An Atlas of
ELECTRONYSTAGMOGRAPHY

An Atlas of
ELECTRONYSTAGMOGRAPHY

by

F. Blair Simmons, M.D.
Division of Otolaryngology
Stanford University Medical School
Stanford, California

with

Suzanne F. Gillam
Clinical Audiologist
Stanford University Medical School
Stanford, California

and

Douglas E. Mattox, M.D.
Division of Otolaryngology
University of Texas Medical Center
San Antonio, Texas

GRUNE & STRATTON

A Subsidiary of Harcourt Brace Jovanovich, Publishers
NEW YORK   SAN FRANCISCO   LONDON

Library of Congress Cataloging in Publication Data

Simmons, Francis Blair, 1930—
    An atlas of electronystagmography.

    Bibliography: p. 191
    Includes index.
    1. Electronystagmography—Atlases. 2. Electro-
nystagmography—Cases, clinical reports, statistics.
I. Gillam, Suzanne, joint author. II. Mattox,
Douglas E., joint author. III. Title.
[DNLM: 1. Electronystagmography—Atlases. WW17
S592a]
RE748.S55   617.7′62′0754   79-1222
ISBN 0-8089-1154-6

Grune & Stratton, Inc.
111 Fifth Avenue
New York, New York 10003

Distributed in the United Kingdom by
Academic Press, Inc. (London) Ltd.
24/28 Oval Road, London NW 1

Library of Congress Catalog Number 79-1222
International Standard Book Number 0-8089-1154-6

Printed in the United States of America

CONTENTS

—

PREFACE

This atlas contains at least one example of every important abnormality recorded by electronystagmography (ENG) during 8000 tests. It also contains a liberal sample of the test artifacts we have encountered since these, too, are part of the clinical milieu when testing patients with symptoms of spatial disorientation. Each patient's clinical history and physical findings are included as a background to complement the ENGs. Some have firm diagnoses and others are obscure. Nearly all have at least a two-year follow-up history.

Each case concludes with a comment on interpretation, reasons for including the ENG, alternative clinical interpretations, and errors in the tracing. These comments are largely in keeping with the current and commonly accepted practice of most electronystagmographers. Sometimes, however, there are differences in opinion or no really well-documented explanations. In these instances I have felt free to offer my own opinions based upon 15 years of clinical experience.

The reader of this atlas will soon discover that the clinical features do not always fit with the classically described ENG abnormalities. Indeed, this is one of the major purposes in selecting the atlas format for this book. Many patients do not fit classical descriptions in textbooks or the periodical literature. Most authors quite understandably tend to present the "ideal" examples of ENG abnormalities and their most common causes, largely because of space limitations. Reproducing the entire ENG allows the student to see abnormalities within the context of the entire tracing. Furthermore, since the normal and abnormal are not identified on the reproductions themselves but only in the text, the readers have the opportunity to make these decisions for themselves, just as they must in clinical practice. Used in this way, the atlas provides considerable clinical experience. Indeed, this atlas began as a series of ENGs collected for teaching our students the process of reading and interpreting ENGs.

The specific abnormalities themselves are liberally indexed and critically referenced both by comments in the text and by references. Thus, the reader who wishes to review the varieties or clinical causes of gaze nystagmus, for example, can do so by using the index.

Two introductory chapters on biophysics and the methods we use in performing the ENG are intended both as background for the beginning student of ENG, and as an introduction to the ENG wholemounts themselves since test methods differ slightly from one laboratory to another. These slight differences, as we point out in these chapters, can have important consequences for the final product.

The ENGs themselves are reduced by about 1:3 from their original size. The quality of the reproductions, however, is very adequate for reading without enlarging except in a few instances. Supplemental enlargements of those segments are provided. An opaque projector can be used to enlarge the entire tracing for greater detail or for group study.

F. Blair Simmons, M.D.

vii

INTRODUCTION

Administering and interpreting electronystagmo-grams (ENGs) are reasonably easy tasks—after the first 500. The major purpose of this atlas is to provide some background for reading those first 500. We have done this by reproducing the complete ENGs of patients, which reflect nearly every abnormality and artifact encountered in over 8000 tests. The worth of these complete records (wholemounts) is that the abnormalities are preserved within the clinical framework of the entire examination. A large part of interpreting an ENG is putting the whole together, not just viewing preselected segments. The task of an ENG interpreter is to detect the normal from the abnormal and the significant from the insignificant. Reviewing the entire tracing is the only way to do this.

Each ENG was selected for specific reasons. These reasons include not only pathological responses but also testing artifacts and errors and even patients who seemingly fall asleep. We have thus tried to keep the theme aimed at practicality and a realistic picture of reading ENGs.

Please take special note that the ENGs were selected first, and then the clinical information was obtained. Thus, these patients do not always have a clear clinical diagnosis. This approach is quite different from one in which tracings are selected by clinical diagnosis. (Presumably, patients undergoing an ENG examination do so *in search of* a diagnosis, not to illustrate further an already established pathology.) One very positive result of selecting the ENGs first is an occasional encounter with a highly abnormal ENG that does not fit the patient's clinical status. This happens often enough in routine testing but is rarely reported in the periodical or textbook literature. It is difficult in such formats to report instances where the patient's illness (if any) does not correspond with the laboratory data. There are several such instances herein, which will serve as a reminder that the ENG itself can only be part of the diagnostic process.

Each ENG is accompanied by a brief clinical history and the more important positive or negative physical findings. We were able to obtain at least a two-year follow-up on nearly all the patients. When a diagnosis is included, it is accurate. We chose not to guess when no diagnosis was clearly established.

While this atlas can be used as a basic ENG text, the patient-oriented format does not flow smoothly from one topic area to the next. Visual suppression of vestibular nystagmus, for example, is mentioned in seven ENGs and is a discussion topic in three of these. We chose not to include basic and essential background material on anatomy and neuro-physiology. We recommend that the reader do some systematic background reading in conjunction with this atlas, if only to gain a different perspective. Quite good and more systematic reviews of ENGs can be found in references 3, 5, 10, 19, 26, and 27.

There are considerable differences in attitudes about electronystagmography. The ENG is not the most accurate way to detect eye motions. In our view, however, it is clearly the most efficient and effective method in the clinical setting for physicians interested in the vestibular system and its interactions with the visual and postural-motor systems. Electronystagmography has its problems and its benefits. It also has its proponents and opponents. Neuro-ophthalmologists, for example, usually do not favor the use of ENGs. Hoyt and Walsh, in their classic 2600-page encyclopedia of neuro-ophthalmology, devote only three paragraphs to electronystagmography.[45] These highly qualified specialists believe they can do a better job by their own visual observations, aided occasionally by Frensel's lens. They can. But they miss things, too, such as changes with closed lids, positional influences, responses to caloric stimulations, arousal phenomena, permanent records, and so on.

READING THE ATLAS

The background material on administering and interpreting an ENG should at least be briefly reviewed by every reader. What appears on the tracings depends heavily on the way the test is administered and on the quality of the recording apparatus. Another laboratory's ENGs may seem different than ours, and the probable reasons are likely to be found in these chapters.

The atlas can be used in one of two ways. The index can be used by the reader interested in a specific abnormality. All important examples of that abnormality are listed. The reader interested in gaining interpretive experience should avoid the index, however, and begin with the first ENG (normal examination) and proceed in order for the next several ENGs. After the first few ENGs, the more difficult and the easier tracings are left unsorted, just as patients are random in their presentations of pathology and symptoms. We strongly advise you not to read the text first. Study the wholemount first. Decide what you think is wrong, and then review the case history and other data.

F. Blair Simmons, M.D.

An Atlas of
ELECTRONYSTAGMOGRAPHY

1.

BIOPHYSICS

The most convenient method for detecting small eye motions is by recording the electrical field changes created by the eye's electrical dipole. This dipole, as diagrammed in Fig. 1-1, is created by a direct current (DC) potential between the retina and the cornea—the corneoretinal potential. The electrical field so created extends outward from the globe for several centimeters. An electrode placed within this field will reflect this voltage. Eye movement causes a change in this voltage which is nearly linearly proportional to the degree of movement. For example, 1° of visual arc movement produces an average of about 10 μv at an electrode placed about 1 cm lateral to the outer canthus. Ten degrees of motion creates a 100-μv potential difference. By ENG convention, the recording electrodes are arranged so that eye movement to the right causes an upward movement of the pen recorder; eye movement to the left, a downward deflection (horizontal electrodes); eye movement upwards, an upward deflection, and so forth (vertical electrodes).

While this retinal voltage is predictably present, it is not a large voltage and can quite easily get buried in the biological electrical noise of the head (muscle contractions, EEG, ECG, and changes in skin resistance). Several technical strategies are very necessary to eliminate or reduce these artifacts.

The first of these, *differential input amplification*, reduces unwanted electrical events generated at comparatively large distances for the eyes. The most common of these are electromagnetic radiations in the atmosphere (60-Hz line voltage radiations; sparks from electrical relay contacts; and sometimes in hospitals, the telepage systems) and ECG activity. In this amplification system, two active electrodes are used instead of one. Typically, for horizontal eye motions, they are placed at both outer canthi but could just as easily be placed at the outer and inner canthi of a single eye. A neutral or ground electrode is placed halfway between these two active electrodes, typically on the forehead, although any other spot halfway in between would do as well. Halfway is the critical feature so that the electrical resistances are equal or nearly equal.

The input stage of the ENG amplifier is constructed for differential amplification of the signals arriving from the two electrodes, both of which are referenced to the same neutral electrode. Only signals that are different at the two electrodes will be amplified. Thus, if the eyes move to the right, the right electrode will have an increasingly negative voltage whereas the left-eye electrode will have an increasingly positive voltage (eye moving toward one electrode and away from the other). This difference will be amplified. On the other hand, an electrical event such as an ECG wave that comes from a distance will not be amplified because it will arrive at the two electrodes at the same time and voltage. Inputs of ECG to the amplifier will be equal and thus cancel one another.

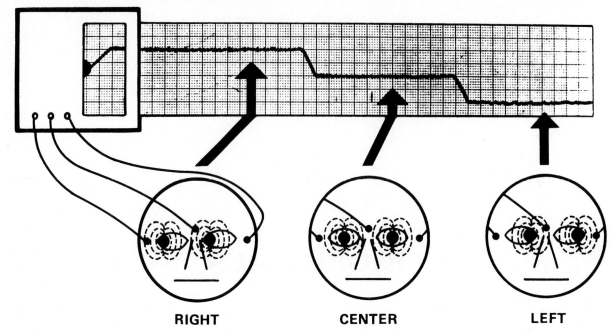

Fig. 1-1. Corneoretinal potential dipole and electrode placement.

High-quality differential amplifiers are capable of rejecting these simultaneous unwanted signals by ratios as high as 100 dB, in favor of the wanted nonidentical signal, in ideal recording conditions. Recording conditions are not always ideal, however. A difference in the resistances between the two active electrodes and the neutral electrode can sometimes profoundly affect this rejection ratio. Recall Ohm's law: the voltage at one electrode is proportional to the resistance between it and the reference point. Thus, if the resistance is greatly higher or lower between one of the two active electrodes and the neutral electrode, there will be an important voltage difference too, and the signal seen by the amplifier will not be equal. No amplifier is adequate to the task of overcoming a poorly applied electrode.

The techniques of differential amplification do not entirely suppress signals that are generated closer to the active electrodes (local muscle noise and EEG). Both of these voltages are much more of a problem when using vertical electrodes where one electrode is anatomically closer to the generators than the other. This is demonstrated on ENGs in this atlas. Eye blinking is the most common of these problems.

High input impedance is another necessary feature of the ENG amplifier. Recall that the eyes' actual voltage on the skin where it is available for electrode pickup is in the microvolt range, that is, a very small voltage. Furthermore, the globe's dipole, which produces this voltage, generates very little current. Thus if we want to tap this voltage with electrodes, the sample of electrons we remove must be minute. If we take a large sample the voltage would drop to near zero (Ohm's law again: voltage = current/resistance). A comparable situation might be an attempt to measure the temperature of a drop of water by using an ordinary thermometer. The initial mass and temperature of the thermometer would affect the water far more than the reverse.

The input resistance (impedance) to the ENG amplifier is therefore deliberately made very high, typically at least 1,000,000 ohms and higher. Thus, very little of the corneoretinal energy will be used by the amplifier. A rough calculation using Ohm's law (assuming the eye's current flow resistance pathway to be about 3000 ohms) yields a ratio of 3000:1,000,000 or 1:333 in favor of the electrons remaining in the biological circuit. The skin resistance also affects this ratio.

Although these high input resistances are essential, they also add problems. Since such small voltages can be amplified, any stray small voltage in the vicinity will also be amplified. The electrode wire and the attached patient both act as antennae to collect these voltages. Furthermore, even movements of the wire strands in the electrode cable can create an adequate small voltage to interfere with a recording. If one or two of these strands are broken, even more electrical noise results (even though an electrode may seem good, try a new one if the ENG recording is noisy). Most of the stray voltages in the atmosphere are at radiofrequencies and are removed by filtering and by the pen recorder itself because it cannot respond to frequencies much above 100 Hz (laboratory-quality recorders can go higher). Only 60-Hz line current is a consistent problem. Most of these radiations should be eliminated either by filtering or by the differential amplifier. Differential amplification continues to work more effectively when the electrode leads are kept symmetrical (together) all the way to the amplifier input. When these precautions have been taken, we have never found it necessary to use special rooms or electrode cable shielding to avoid line voltage interference.

Alternating current (AC) amplification rather than DC amplification is used by most ENG laboratories to avoid the major artifacts and baseline changes that occur with changes in the patients' skin resistance. An individual's skin resistance can change rapidly by at least several hundred ohms and for a variety of reasons that cannot be controlled. These changes induce sizable voltages into the recording system and are often large enough to throw the pen completely off the edge of the strip chart for seconds or minutes. One way to prevent this is to limit the low-frequency sensitivity of the amplifier. In this way, any slowly changing voltage will not be amplified, and the pen stays on the paper.

The disadvantage of low-frequency filtering is that the record will no longer register a sustained tonic deviation of the eye. Consider, as in Fig. 1-2, the DC recording of a tonic 10-second eye deviation (dashed line). The AC recording (solid line) would achieve the same initial deflection but decay toward the baseline according to the setting of the low-frequency filter, its time constant.

The *time constant* is thus always a compromise between coming as close to direct current as possible without the amplifier accepting minor skin resistance changes as a signal. The value most commonly used is 3 seconds. This constant is used by most, if not all, manufacturers of ENG machines and is also available as a choice on machines that are capable of DC recording. Unfortunately, our experience has shown that manufacturers' concepts of a 3-second time constant can differ widely. Furthermore, machines in use can lose their calibration.[40] Time constants that are less than about 3 seconds cause the pen to decay to the baseline too rapidly. While this may make the ENG tracing look more even, too much detail of eye motions can be lost as well as creating inaccurate estimates of the eye's movement velocity.

A rough estimate of the time constant of an ENG machine is available on the ENG tracing during gaze testing. The tonic eye deviation of 30° will produce enough of a change in the DC potential to

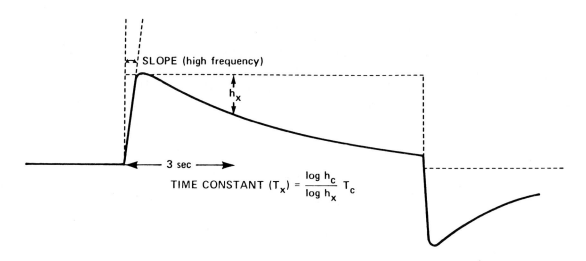

$$\text{TIME CONSTANT } (T_x) = \frac{\log h_c}{\log h_x}\, T_c$$

Fig. 1-2. Alternating current versus direct current recording — frequency response for a 10-second pulse.

cause the pen to swing off or nearly off the paper (see ENG 1 for an example). During the right-gaze test in particular, the pen deflects off the paper and then decays gradually toward the baseline at a rate determined by the low-frequency sensitivity of the machine. The initial 30° deflection upwards (right gaze) is also one place to check on the high-frequency limits of the recorder. The pen should be able to follow a 30° deflection as easily as the 10° calibration.

High-frequency filtering is really unnecessary as a strategy to get good-quality ENG tracings, except at 60 Hz. All the office-type heat stylus recorders are, in fact, incapable of responding linearly beyond 7 Hz, and most yield very poor quality tracings at pen speeds of 5 Hz. Ink and electric writing recorders have much better capabilities, with speeds of 20 Hz and above. These units are more expensive and are seldom found outside hospital or institutional settings. These machines do a better job of registering the fine detail of eye motions.

GROUND LOOPS

The elimination of all possible current pathways except the desired one from the patient is an important safety and interference-reducing consideration. The elimination of unanticipated current flow pathways is not always easy and comes as close to being a black art as anything the author has encountered in electronics. Anything that can go wrong will do so eventually. Major ground loops of the type capable of carrying damaging amounts of current will not be reviewed here. Barber and Stockwell do a fine job of discussing these considerations.[5]

The more minor but severely frustrating ground loops are those that cause 60-Hz interference no matter how faithfully the electrodes are applied and other precautions taken. The patient-to-ENG-amplifier part of the system operates at a very high electrical resistance above ground. An electron in the high-resistance part of the system will try to get to ground the easiest way it can and will seek out any lower resistance pathway in the vicinity. If it finds one, it flows (current), and this will appear as 60 Hz on the recording.

All possible alternatives to ground can be eliminated by connecting all equipment, and any other substantial pieces of metal in the room, to a common ground. Do not assume, for example, that the grounding pins of all line voltage receptacles in the room are connected to an identical ground. If more than one receptacle is used, measure all the grounding pins against one another with a voltmeter. There should be no recordable reading on maximum scale. Also measure the maximum scale voltage between the different pieces of equipment in the room. These, too, should read zero when turned on and operating. If not, it is time to call for consultation.

ELECTRODE-SKIN INTERFACE

The most critical recurring problem for beginners using ENG machines is the electrode-skin interface. There are at least three elements that have important and dynamic influences on the quality and precision of eye-movement recordings—the skin, the electrolyte paste, and the electrode itself. Careful attention to all three will keep the resistance to tapping the corneoretinal potential at a minimum.

The skin site selected for electrode application should be as close to the orbit as possible but far enough away so as not to be affected by the skin and muscle motion of blinks and other lid movements.

For horizontal electrodes, a placement about 1½ cm lateral to the outer canthus is usually satisfactory. Vertical electrodes are more of a placement problem because the fibers of the orbicularis muscle sometimes extend 2 cm below the orbit, and the frontalis muscle cannot be avoided in placing the upper electrode. The reference or ground electrode should be placed in the midline, preferably as high on the forehead as possible, to reduce muscle artifacts. The tip of the nose is a good alternative if the forehead cannot be used. The normal skin resistance in ideal circumstances varies between 2000 and 5000 ohms. The lower this resistance is, the better. All superficial skin debris and oily substances must be removed with vigorous enthusiasm. A fat solvent such as alcohol or acetone is used.

The electrolyte paste serves to reduce the resistance between the skin and the electrode. The ion composition of all commercially available ECG or EEG paste is adequate for ENG application. The viscosity is important, however, since a solution that is too thin is likely to spread over an area larger than the electrode and thereby reduce the accuracy of the recording. Thin solutions also increase the likelihood of muscle and motion artifacts. Apply just enough paste to fit under the electrode. The skin-electrolyte junction is never completely stable, but most of the variability in resistance occurs in the first 5 minutes as the solution penetrates and moistens the superficial layers of the skin. It is thus wise to *wait 5 minutes after the electrodes have been applied before beginning the ENG.*

There are two basic types of electrodes in general use, the standard EEG-type electrode and an electrode originally designed for DC recording. The EEG electrodes are considerably less expensive but cannot be used in DC application because of some rather complicated and poorly understood electrochemical reactions at the boundary of the electrolyte and the metal. Since the ions in the metal and those in the electrolyte are different, an ion boundary layer develops at this junction. This produces a voltage gradient or junction potential. A direct current cannot pass this ion barrier unless its voltage exceeds that of the junction. The junction potential varies among electrolyte and metal combinations but is typically 0.2 to 1 mv, much larger than the corneoretinal potential under the electrode.

If DC records are desired, this junction potential can be considerably attenuated by pretreating the electrode surface with the ion in the electrolyte solution so that a chemical bond is formed on the surface. The most common of these is a silver electrode, deposited with chloride ions to form a silver-silver chloride layer. This layer is both light-sensitive and highly unstable. A new chloride application is required at frequent intervals. The Beckman Company manufactures a clever compromise electrode in which replaceable pellets of AgCl are used. These are held off the skin and in contact with the electrolyte by a plastic cap.

Either type of electrode must be firmly fixed on the skin to minimize movement. This connection should be rigid enough to withstand a healthy tug. Movement of the electrode during recording produces a sizable voltage. Plastic tape or precut circular patches are the adhesives commonly used.

ENG RECORDERS

Although there are no formal standards maintained for ENG recorders as there are for audiometers, certain characteristics are common to most. Some of these have been mentioned in the preceding pages. Purchase decisions are most frequently based upon other features, such as number of channels, type of writer (ink, heat, electrical), paper costs, and frequency of use. As elsewhere, you get what you pay for. Nearly everyone who performs a large number of ENGs and those who are considered to be the "experts" in the field use general-purpose strip-chart recorders with ink-writing styli, rather than machines marketed as "ENG machines." The general-purpose recorders are more expensive but cost less in paper and breakdown time to operate. They also have better frequency responses, more paper speeds, and more options on numbers of channels. The majority of office-type ENG machines should be suitable for test situations where the patient volume does not justify the expense of a more elegant system. Some (about half in the author's experience) of these machines develop such poor response characteristics after a time that one would be hesitant to use them as a clinical diagnostic aid.

Number of Channels

Ninety-nine percent of the time, a single recording channel is quite adequate. A second or third channel is largely a convenience in most instances, used either to record the electrically integrated slow or fast phase of a nystagmus or as a spare channel in case the first breaks down. We have not found simultaneous recording of both the horizontal and vertical vector of eye motion sufficiently rewarding to use routinely. We do so only when visual observation or the patient's specific symptoms seem to indicate using vertical electrodes. A single-channel unit can record both, but not simultaneously.

Paper Speed

A paper speed of 5 mm/sec is quite adequate for almost all applications. Most ENG machines have a 10 mm/sec paper drive, and although this is certainly acceptable, it uses twice as much paper. A nice luxury is a multispeed paper drive with 1, 5, and 25 mm/sec capability. The faster paper speed is sometimes essential to resolve the characteristics of very rapid eye motions. The slower speed can be used during caloric irrigations to detect onset time differences between a tactilely induced or accentuated spontaneous nystagmus and a true response to the caloric stimuli.

Gain and Sensitivity

The recorder's sensitivity—the index of the smallest signal it will amplify—is really indexed by two numbers, the internal electrical noise of the amplifiers and the millimeters of pen deflection produced by an input signal that is slightly greater than the noise floor of the amplifier. It is reasonable to expect a 1-mm pen deflection per each 2-μv increment in the input signal and a noise level of 7 μv or less. Calibration of eye movement for a standard pen deflection requires a continuously variable gain control. A nice luxury is a second gain control with fixed settings at one-half and at twice the variable gain setting. This control allows the operator to reduce or increase the pen swings without having to recalibrate the system. This feature is most useful in recording very rapid caloric-induced nystagmus.

Direct Current Versus Alternating Current

A recorder capable of operating in the DC mode is almost always superior to one limited to AC. All DC recorders also have AC capabilities. They are also more expensive. Very few clinical electronystagmographers use DC recording, however. In the author's opinion, it is completely unnecessary. Yet because of the better electrical stability that must be built into the DC machine, a DC machine used in the AC mode is recommended.

2.

TESTING PROCEDURE

Our testing order is the same as that described in the following paragraphs. There is nothing sacred about this order except that it must end with caloric stimulation. All segments except optokinetic testing are performed with the patient lying down, usually with a 30° head elevation. The room is dimly illuminated except during the visual tests. Other laboratories perform many of these tests with the patient sitting. We do this, too, occasionally and have found no important differences.

APPLICATION OF ELECTRODES

We use standard EEG disc electrodes. The two active electrodes (horizontal eye motion) are applied about 1½ cm lateral to each outer canthus. In some individuals, it is necessary to place the electrodes slightly farther from the eye to avoid muscle and motion artifacts. The reference or ground electrode is placed in the center of the forehead (Fig. 2-1). Electrodes for recording vertical eye motion are placed above and below the center axis of the globe, just beyond the fibers of the orbicularis muscle. There is considerable variability among individuals in the perimetry of this muscle, especially below the eye. Blink artifacts and muscle motion will heavily contaminate vertical recordings, even with "good" placements. It may take one or two reapplications to obtain satisfactory tracings.

The skin is first vigorously cleaned with a fat solvent such as alcohol. The skin should be scrubbed hard enough to remove the superficial layer of dead epithelial cells. A viscous-type EEG paste is then applied to the electrode disc. We use just enough paste to ensure that the electrode will not be in contact with the skin (Fig. 2-2). (An alternative is to use just enough paste to ensure that the electrode will always be in contact with the skin. The important point is to guard against intermittent skin-electrode contact because such irregular contacts cause very large voltage-change artifacts.) The electrodes are then placed firmly and secured with two pieces of plastic tape. The tape should also secure the first centimeter or two of the lead wire.

We then wait at least 5 minutes before beginning the ENG. This waiting period is usually sufficient to reach electrical equilibrium between the skin potentials, the paste penetration, and the electrode-paste interface.

Comment

Competent ENG recordings cannot be obtained without scrupulous concern for proper electrode placement and mechanical (motion) stability. Poor

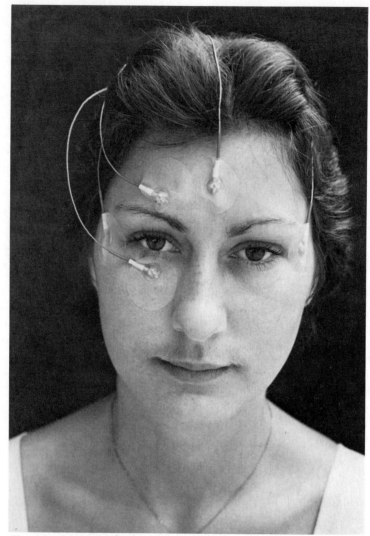

Fig. 2-1. Locations for horizontal, vertical, and reference electrodes.

technique causes more interpretive problems than any other variable except the patient's level of arousal. It takes time, effort, and experience to apply the electrodes properly. The first thing to check if the recording seems bizarre is the electrodes. Never hesitate to refix or replace an electrode. Wires break inside the insulation casing and cannot be seen.

CALIBRATION

The gain of the recorder must be adjusted so that 10° of lateral (or vertical) eye motion causes 10 mm of pen deflection. This calibration must be done several times throughout the test for each patient because there is considerable variability among patients and in the same patient at different times. By convention, the electrodes should be arranged so that a deviation to the right (or upwards with vertical electrodes) causes an upward pen movement and deviation to the left causes a downward movement. We use two calibration targets 10° apart. Other laboratories use three calibrations 10° to the right and left of a center target.

The calibration targets should be at least 2 meters

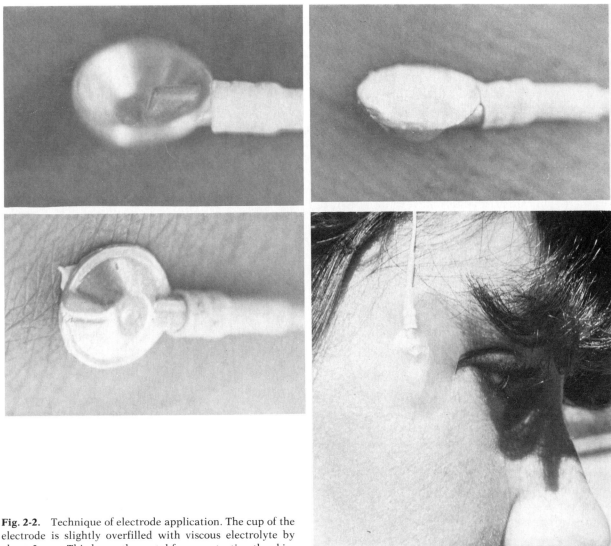

Fig. 2-2. Technique of electrode application. The cup of the electrode is slightly overfilled with viscous electrolyte by about 2 mm. This keeps the metal from contacting the skin. The electrode is then fastened firmly to the skin by either plastic tape or precut circular adhesive patches.

from the patient's eyes. The distance between the targets subtending 10° of visual arc can be determined by trigonometric formulas or just as easily by measuring the distance, multiplying by 2 × 3.14, and dividing by 36. This number will be 10°.

Calibrations are also an important part of the ENG test itself and can yield considerable diagnostic information if properly done. The patients are asked to fixate on the "on" light as the tester alternately switches from right to left while adjusting the recorder gain. It is important not to automate the switching from one target to another if you are planning to use the calibration tracking as part of the diagnostic battery. If the alternation is regular,

patients can be rapidly conditioned to anticipate the target switch rather than track it. Bright, pinpoint light sources should be used.* The pinpoint lights are not only easy to see but also much easier for the patient to maintain in steady gaze. Fixation on pinpoint lights is partially a reflex act, whereas looking at a mark on the wall is entirely volitional and will not give the same results. Some patients have trouble seeing the targets. The use of eyeglasses is acceptable. Calibrations with blind persons can be

---

* We use flashlight bulbs, powered by line voltage through a transformer. The pinpoint is created by covering the bulbs with the rubber end of a medicine dropper that has a small hole in it.

done by asking them to "track" the position of their thumb as the tester moves it through 10° of arc.

It is not always possible to attain 10 mm of pen deflection. Some elderly patients and others with retinal disorders have reduced corneoretinal voltages.[31] Proceed anyway, but take this difference into account later when calculating eye velocities.

Dark adaptation can also affect this voltage, and some authors have claimed this to be an important variable. We have never found this to be true in clinical practice. Probably the largest swings in calibration are caused by changes in patients' skin resistance, and these can easily halve or double during the progress of the test. Therefore, we calibrate many times—at the beginning, after the positioning tests, and immediately after each caloric.

A precisely used calibration can yield considerable technical and clinical information.[21] ENGs 13, 16, 17, 26, 36 and 37 show some examples. The test is also the best place to look for built-in artifacts in your own recordings and in recordings from unfamiliar laboratories. The most common of these is the recorder with a very poor response to high frequencies. Heat stylus machines are particularly susceptible. The right-left peaks are rounded like the example shown in Figure 2-3B. This will also cause nystagmus beats to seem rounded, small degrees of gaze nystagmus or fixation nystagmus to be missed completely, and falsely low values of nystagmus velocity among other sins. If the right-left deflections are rounded in only one direction (Fig. 2-3C), there may be either a unilateral uneven pen pressure on the paper or a defect in one-half of the ENG amplifier.

Poor low-frequency responses (short time constant) are also common. In fact, some laboratories deliberately use short time constants to help keep the tracing centered on the paper. This strategy may produce a neater product, but the need to do so may also hide other defects in the testing system, such as poorly applied electrodes. Figure 2-3D is an example. The tracing drops rapidly toward the baseline. The defect will cause the ENG reader dif-

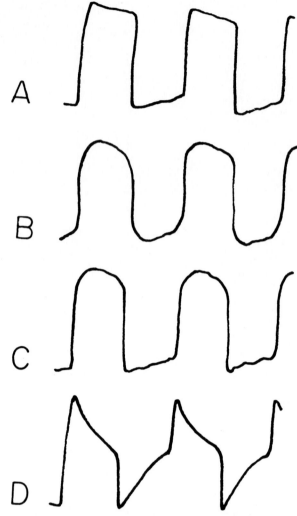

Fig. 2-3. Calibration defects caused by ENG machine malfunctions. (A) Normal calibration. (B) Poor high-frequency response. (C) Uneven pen pressure on paper or a faulty amplifier. (D) Poor low-frequency response (short time constant).

ficulty in detecting tonic deviation of the eyes, in seeing slow nystagmus velocities, and in differentiating rhythmic eye blinks from nystagmus and will cause slow-phase velocity distortions.[40]

GAZE TESTING

In gaze testing (Fig. 2-4), we ask the patient to fixate on a pencil or similar object held about 50 cm away. The head is in the primary or midline position. Gaze is tested with the eyes centered and at no more than 30° to the left and right. Each position is maintained for 15 to 20 seconds. Most persons have some degree of end-point nystagmus when lateral gaze exceeds 30°, which is at about the point where the edge of the iris meets the lateral canthus (Fig. 2-4C).

It is important for the tester to observe these eye

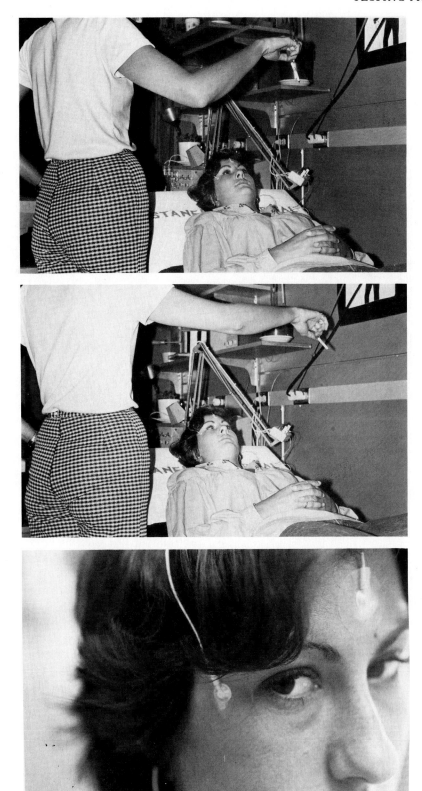

Fig. 2-4. Gaze testing. (A) Eyes center, with fixation. (B) Eyes left. (C) Eyes right at approximately 30° (edge of iris at lateral canthus).

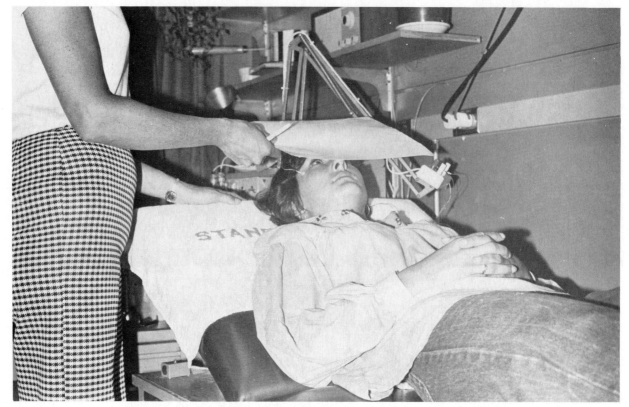

Fig. 2-5. Eyes open, no fixation.

motions. The ENG cannot record a muscle imbalance or paralysis, glass eyes, minor convergence nystagmus, or other asymmetrical eye motions. These defects are essential to note for the total ENG analysis later on.

Eyes Open, No Fixation

In the eyes-open, no-fixation procedure (Fig. 2-5), the patient is asked to continue center gaze. Fixation is prevented by placing a plain white cardboard within 3 inches of the eyes for about 20 seconds. This is an important baseline test, both for comparison with types of visual nystagmus accentuated by fixation and for vestibular nystagmus which is inhibited both by fixation and by the presence of light without fixation.

Eyes Closed, Head

The eyes-closed, head-center procedure is the final transition from a visually dominated set of eye movements to movements dominated by the vestibular system (Fig. 2-6). This typically is the first time that a vestibular pathway spontaneous nystagmus is observed. Some nystagmus has an onset latency of 30 to 40 seconds, and recording should continue for at least 40 seconds.

Random changes (saccades) in the baseline may skyrocket once the lids are closed. Although these random eye motions sometimes produce a messy tracing, we like to see these saccades because they indicate that the patient is alert. Once the lids are closed, alertness can be a problem, so begin making certain that the patient is wide awake and thinking. Some anxious patients have excessive eye blinking or lid flutter which interferes with recording nystagmus. This can be reduced by placing your fingers lightly on the closed eyelids. Light or even slightly heavy pressure will not affect nystagmus.

Positional Effects

While the lids are still closed, the patient is asked to rotate his head to an extreme right lateral position for at least 40 seconds, then to the left, and then

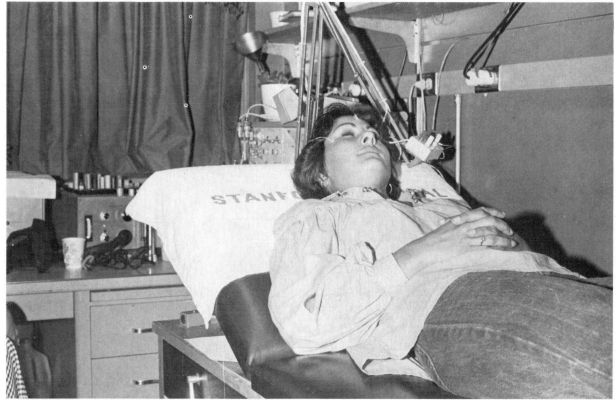

Fig. 2-6. Eyes closed, head center.

to hyperextend the head for a similar amount of time (Fig. 2-7). If either lateral maneuver produces nystagmus or has an obvious effect on a spontaneous (head-center) nystagmus, we also test for neck torsion effects by asking the patient to lie on his right and left sides, thus avoiding neck rotation. If any of these maneuvers accentuate or produce symptoms, it is noted on the recording.

We do not perform the classical head-hanging maneuvers of Hallpike during routine ENG testing unless the patient is specifically symptomatic in such positions. This test has not been particularly valuable for us on a routine basis and is probably best left to the examining physician to perform. Harrison has written an excellent review of this test.[22]

OPTOKINETIC (OPN or OKN) TESTING

For OPN testing (Figure 2-8), we use a three-speed motor-driven black and white striped drum which is large enough to accommodate the patient's head inside. The patient is instructed to "look at the stripes" at at least two drum speeds if the first response is abnormal. The speeds are approximately 15° and 30° of visual arc per second. Exact rates differ slightly because the distance between the patient's eyes and the drum surface varies.

This is an easy task for most patients. They do use slightly different strategies in following the stripes. Some pursue a stripe for 30° off the midline, and others deviate only a few degrees before refixing on the next white-black entering their field of vision. Some persons are very exact and match the rotations of the drum precisely. Others lag in their eye movements and move their eyes more slowly than the drum rotates. Both are normal. Abnormal behavior is usually obvious—a complete inability to track rotations in one direction or in both direc-

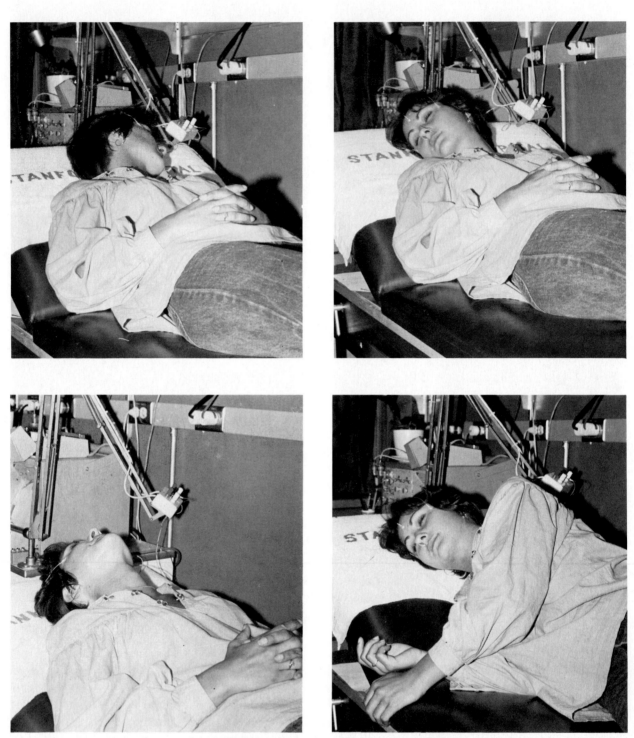

Fig. 2-7. Positional testing. (A) Head left. (B) Head right. (C) Head back. (D) Body rotation without neck torsion.

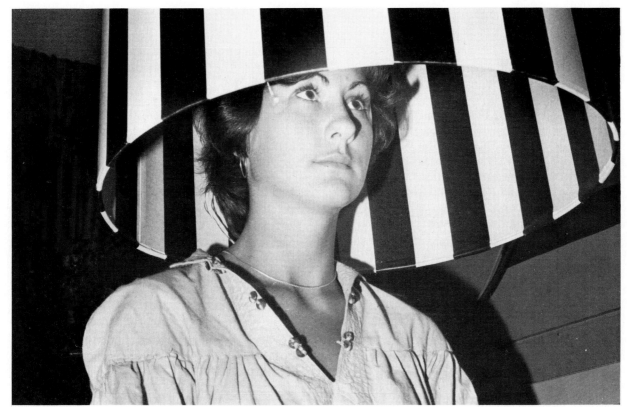

Fig. 2-8. Optokinetic test.

tions. Bilaterally poor performers may need to be reinstructed or otherwise encouraged to "try harder" before assuming an abnormality.

We use horizontal OPN only for routine testing. Some clinics also test OPN in the vertical plane. The additional diagnostic yield from vertical OPN is minimal.

We also sometimes use a moving light to test pursuit movements. The authors do not believe this piece of equipment is necessary or often very helpful in diagnoses. A simple pendulum would do as well in producing a sinusoidal motion for the patient to track.

CALORICS

The nominal goal of causing temperature-induced endolymph flow in the semicircular canals is to test their function, using nystagmus as the readout. If the end-organs and reflex pathways are all normal, equal thermal stimuli in each ear will cause equal amounts of nystagmus. The resulting nystagmus is mainly in the horizontal plane because the horizontal canals are maximally affected (perhaps 95 percent) by conventional clinical head positioning of these canals in the vertical plane.

Warm water (typically 7°C above body temperature) causes endolymph flow upwards or toward the vestibule and ampula and a tonic deviation of the eyes toward the opposite side. An unfortunate custom dictates, however, that the direction of a nystagmus is the direction of the compensatory (quick or saccadic) phase, which is to the same side. Cool water produces an opposite reaction of approximately the same magnitude. The warm calorics are probably closer to a normal physiological stimulus than cool irrigations. Most of the body's postural hemostatic mechanisms have their stronger effect on the contralateral half of the body.

Head position is a critical variable during the

measurement of nystagmus. The horizontal semicircular canal must be in the gravitational vertical plane for maximum stimulation. To accomplish this, adjust the patient's head so that the ear canal and outer canthus of the eye are in a vertical plane. Tests administered sitting or lying down are equivalent, just as long as this plane is maintained. Investigators have used other head positionings to stimulate the other two semicircular canals, but these maneuvers have not seen clinical application. For example, a complete 180° rotation of the head (nose-down position) causes the convection currents and the direction of horizontal canal nystagmus to reverse direction completely.

Procedure

We use the conventional Fitzgerald-Hallpike bithermal caloric stimuli at 30° and 44°C.[16] We deliver a large volume of distilled water (typically 240 ml) over a 40-second period. This is automatically timed and stopped. This automation is important because the technician has enough to do in making sure the water is actually entering the ear and collected afterwards besides watching a clock. Minor variations in irrigation temperature are less important than achieving a large volume flow in a measured time. (See the ENG-23 discussion for additional comments.) Some laboratories use a 30-second irrigation period, and this, too, is adequate.

After stimulation, the patient's head is positioned as mentioned above (eyes closed). The ENG machine can be left on during the caloric stimulations but at a very slow speed (1 mm/sec). This is now increased to 5 mm/sec, and nystagmus is recorded either until it stops or for about 3 minutes. An eyes-open no-fixation test is given at about 90 seconds. (The exact interval is not crucial as long as there is still an observable nystagmus with the eyes closed.) If this test is positive (an increased slow-phase velocity with eyes open), it is repeated several times. If an eyes-closed nystagmus is unusually brisk, we reduce the amplifier gain by one-half. This makes it easier to calculate slow-phase velocity later on. (If the form of the nystagmus is unusual, we will sometimes increase the paper speed to 25 mm/sec for a more detailed tracing.) A repeat calibration is done immediately after each caloric, and this calibration is used in the eye-speed calculations. We then wait at least 5 minutes before the next stimulus. If one of the four calorics is markedly different than the other three, that irrigation is then repeated. If the nystagmus is either severely hypoactive or absent, we then use 5 ml of ice water as a maximal test stimulus.

Comments

Ear Examination: An otoscopic examination for excessive wax, infections, and tympanic membrane perforations is an essential preparatory step. Do not assume that the referring physician has had the foresight to underwrite the absence of these conditions. Minor amounts of wax are unimportant and can be overcome by using a high-volume irrigation. Major amounts are good thermal insulators and must be removed. Minor ear canal infections are not an absolute contraindication to caloric irrigations, but the ear canals should be dried thoroughly afterwards, and we follow this with antibiotic ear drops on rare occasions. Perhaps the use of distilled water helps reduce the bacteria count in the covered tanks. A tympanic membrane perforation is a relative contraindication to routine calorics. We use refrigerated antibiotic ear drops instead, unless there is a specific and important reason also to apply a warm stimulus. Alternative methods include irrigation through a finger cot in the ear canal or air calorics. These extremes are rarely, if ever, necessary in search of a clinical diagnosis.

For general use, air calorics are not as effective as water calorics. The range of normal variability is larger, and the precision of directing the airstream is much more critical than water flow. Furthermore, if the ear canal or middle ear in perforated drums is moist, the warm air caloric effect may actually be cancelled because of the cooling effect of evaporation. We do not recommend air calorics for routine stimulation.

Alertness: The major obstacle in obtaining accurate test results is the patients. Lack of alertness is the *major source* of error in caloric tests. Patients get drowsy and they get bored. Some can sleep during the recordings. This fact is not given the emphasis it deserves either in the clinical literature or by laboratories who pay more attention to meticulously adjusting their caloric temperatures to a ±0.1°C precision for increased accuracy. The person who is on the receiving end of all this precision makes the real difference. The patient who is highly aroused or anxious will produce as much as twice the normal nystagmus velocities. The patient who is inattentive will generate half-normal responses, and sometimes even no nystagmus at all. Yet in both states, their real vestibular functions may be entirely normal. If you are unconvinced, try it yourself. Keep yourself aroused and actively thinking (any subject will do) during one caloric and then repeat the caloric while sleepy.

Most individuals can be kept alert by doing mental arithmetic. The answers must be spoken aloud. A common routine is to subtract 7's from 100. Accountants can do this and still get drowsy. Use any mental task that challenges the patient. Be creative, but keep at it during the entire test. Keep the patient thinking and talking.

Arousal has a powerful effect on all phases of the eyes-closed ENG. Decreased arousal can inhibit or attenuate a spontaneous nystagmus, for example. This arousal decrement can be helped along by sedative drugs, too. Sometimes the caloric stimulus itself, by tactile or thermal stimulation of the ear canal, will arouse the patient and reveal a spontaneous nystagmus not recorded earlier. This nystagmus, in the presence of a nonresponsive or severely hypoactive labyrinth, can quite easily be interpreted as a true caloric-induced vestibular nystagmus. This is why we leave the ENG machine running at reduced paper speed while administering the calorics. If a nystagmus begins immediately with the water, it is an arousal effect, not a caloric nystagmus.

Dysrhythmia during calorics is first highly suggestive of arousal effects and can only be judged as a significant abnormality if you are confident that the patient is awake and working. Lack of adequate alertness is the most common cause for an increase in vestibular nystagmus when the eyes are open. A true failure of visual suppression of caloric-induced nystagmus is important as a pathological finding, but it is rare.

Failure of Fixation Suppression (FFS): Our test for FFS during calorics is different from most. In fact, we prevent fixation when asking the patient to open his eyes by placing a sheet of plain white cardboard about 3 inches away. The main reason for this testing difference was subsequently vindicated by Levy et al., who have shown that the pathological nystagmus increment with the eyes-open test is actually the failure of light to suppress the nystagmus, not the ability to fix vision on a target. Visual fixation also inhibits vestibular nystagmus, but by different nervous pathways which are largely uninvolved

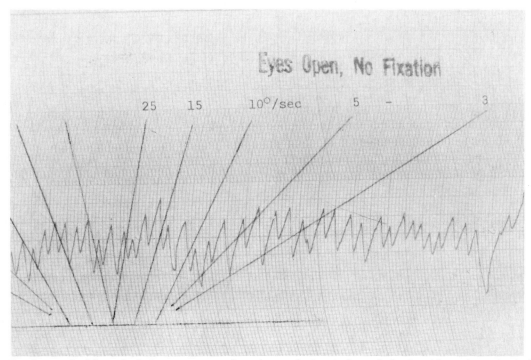

Fig. 2-9. Overlay method for calculating nystagmus slow-phase velocity. A sheet of plastic with predetermined slope lines corresponding to intervals of slow-phase velocity is placed over the ENG. In this example, the velocity is closest to 25° per second.

with the classical FFS test. Thus the presence or absence of light is the major influence on the FFS test. Consider also that some patients have poor vision at best and cannot perform this immensely more complicated task of holding their eyes on a target while feeling dizzy from the caloric stimulus. If you decide to require fixation, make sure the patient can see the target.

The FFS test should only be considered positive if you are certain the patient is alert and if the findings are present on many repeat eye openings. A true positive will be obvious. Do not overread minor velocity changes.

Measurement of Slow-Phase Velocity: Like most other investigators, we use slow-phase velocity as the index for caloric reactivity. Nystagmus begins about 30 seconds after beginning stimulation, reaches maximum between 60 and 90 seconds, and then decays gradually over the next 2 minutes. There is much normal variability in the nystagmus end point. Three minutes of measurement is adequate. In fact, some laboratories compare only the 60- to 90-second segments of their recordings. (This abbreviation is risky for estimating arousal effects, superimposed spontaneous nystagmus, dysmetria, and other more subtle features.) The calibration values taken immediately afterwards are used in calculating slow-phase velocity.

We use a transparent plastic overlay to estimate velocity. The plastic has predetermined line slopes that are matched to the slopes on the tracing. Figure 2-9 illustrates this method. The slow-phase velocity varies by as much as 30 percent from beat to beat in some individuals, so an average of three measurements are taken at 30-second intervals.

The range of normal maximum nystagmus velocities produced by 7°C stimuli varies among laboratories. Aschan et al. report an average of 11° per second and quote Henriksson's average as 29° per second with a ±11° per second variation.[3] Barber and Wright's range is 6° to 80°.[5] Our normal range is about 10° to 35°. Most authors place more emphasis on caloric asymmetry in clinical application. One ear is hypoactive (paretic) when there is a 7 to a 25 percent difference between ears, according to two studies. We tend to agree with Coats, who uses a 30 percent difference in slow-phase velocity as the limit between normal and abnormal right-left symmetry.[10] A nystagmus (directional) preponderance exists when there is a greater than 15 to 29 percent difference between right- and left-going nystagmus.[24] We tend not to read an ENG as showing a nystagmus preponderance unless the difference in the two directions exceeds about 30 percent. Data on velocity variation with age are not available for children, who are notoriously difficult to test, but in adults, there is a gradual increasing responsiveness until 65 years of age and then a decrement.[8]

3.

THE PROCESS OF OBTAINING AND INTERPRETING AN ENG

There is no commonly accepted single method or approach to reading and interpreting an ENG tracing. Some laboratories rely heavily on a technician for interpretation because the physician reviews only those segments of the tracing that have been preselected and mounted by the technician. Others never utilize a technician in any step of the test or its interpretation. This second approach is much to be preferred, particularly in the beginning. But, sooner or later, almost everyone resorts to a technician as the patient volume increases.

Knowing the integrity and competency of the technician is thus the first and most critical step in reading an ENG. The technician must first be able to use an otoscope competently. Administering a good, reliable test is far more demanding than it is with ECGs or EEGs. There must be considerable patient-technician interaction, not only to keep the patient alert and concentrating on the several tasks but also to gain information on medications, body-position-related symptoms, and other bits and pieces of history garnered over the 45 minutes of testing. A disinterested technician or one who is not made to feel that his or her role is part of the entire diagnostic process is not going to get an accurate test. There should always be means for feedback between technician and physician, including not only technical problems but also patient diagnoses and follow-up. Thus the laboratory itself should be within the office or clinic setting where this interaction can take place conveniently. The author knows a number of laboratories where this interaction is lacking, and the result is poor-quality tracings that are frequently inaccurate to the point of complete worthlessness.

Our routine upon the first patient contact is to eliminate all sedative and antihistamine drugs for 3 days before the test. We prefer to mail the patient a list of instructions when possible. Oral instructions, improperly understood, have sometimes led patients to discontinue life-supporting medications in addition to sedatives. It is sometimes necessary to test patients who cannot be completely free of pain medications, and in these instances, a caution about interpretation of the results is always included. Patients taking diphenylhydantoin are a particular problem. We strongly suggest that a blood level be obtained beforehand if possible and always afterwards if certain signs are present in the ENG.

We ask the patient to complete a dizziness questionnaire after arrival for the test. We have found the questionnaire to be helpful in checking for medications and to get the patient thinking about his symptoms in some detail. We have not found the information particularly valuable or accurate as an aid in obtaining a classical history or in interpreting the ENG itself.

After the tracings are obtained, the technician plots the slow phase velocities of the caloric stimulations at 30-second intervals and transmits these and

ENG VESTIBULAR REPORT

(1-10) NAME: _____

(11-16) MEDICAL RECORD # _____

(17-22) DATE: _____

(23-24) AGE: _____

Fig. 3-1. Work sheet used to record ENG findings.

70-47-7 (Rev. 4/77)

the entire uncut tracing to the physician reader. We use a reading report form (Fig. 3-1) whose format is arranged for convenience in transferring the data to keypunch cards. Each box has a corresponding one- or two-sentence descriptor, which, when strung together, generates the written report without the reader doing so each time an ENG is read. About 5 percent of ENGs require some additional written comment.

The completed form and the ENG are returned to the technician, who then mounts selected segments of the tracing (Figs. 3-2, 3-3, and 3-4), and completes the written report that accompanies the mounted segments.

In reading these ENGs, we usually deliberately avoid any attempt at a clinical diagnosis. Our laboratory accepts patients from any physician who requests an ENG. The ENG is only a laboratory test, no different in function than ordering a white blood count. It is not the laboratory's mission to provide a clinical diagnosis—only information that may or may not be helpful in arriving at a diagnosis. We do not require nor really want a clinical history but prefer to read the tracing without any additional information that might bias objectivity. The written report concludes with the statement normal, abnormal, or borderline and then lists the abnormalities. We will sometimes also include a comment on clinical relevance if the abnormalities completely indicate a specific locale or problem or if the ENG has something quite unusual about it that the referring physician might otherwise overlook.

The most common error in ENG interpretation is a tendency to overread the tracing. This tendency is particularly prevalent in persons new to the process who have just invested considerable time and money in establishing a laboratory and who may subconsciously need to justify this effort by uncovering each and every possible diagnostic crumb from the first few records. Avoid this tendency first by testing some normal subjects, including at least

two children 6 to 8 years old. Second, if you cannot see the abnormality in the tracing from at least 6 feet away, with one eye closed and the other squinting, it probably does not exist.

Expect at least 50 percent of the ENGs to be normal. We get a little uneasy when the number of abnormal ENGs rises much beyond 50 percent for a month or two. If the test is being administered properly and read consistently, a high rate of abnormals probably means that it is being used in a suboptimal manner as a diagnostic tool. That is, patients undergoing ENG testing already have a fairly solid clinical diagnosis to which the abnormal ENG adds little new information.

There are differences of opinion about the division between a normal and an abnormal ENG. Perhaps the best, though least important, example of this are the large variations in normal caloric-induced nystagmus obtained from different established laboratories. Not all variables in the test are under quite as good control as one would suppose from reading the literature. Other normal–abnormal borderlines that can cause interpretive problems are small amounts of spontaneous or positional nystagmus, caloric dysmetria, asymmetrical but not dysmetric OPNs, and visual tracking tasks. Some interpreters take a very hard line, for example, and consider as normal all spontaneous nystagmus with velocities of less than 6° per second. The logic applied is that some "normal" individuals have this amount of nystagmus (sometimes more) and yet have no symptoms. We disagree with this philosophy and in theory consider any nystagmus abnormal. We do agree, however, that while abnormal, it may not be clinically significant and may be totally irrelevant to the patient's problem. In such instances, our overall impression of an ENG might be borderline normal or borderline abnormal instead of normal or abnormal. Some of these borderline abnormalities will be reviewed in the ENGs later on.

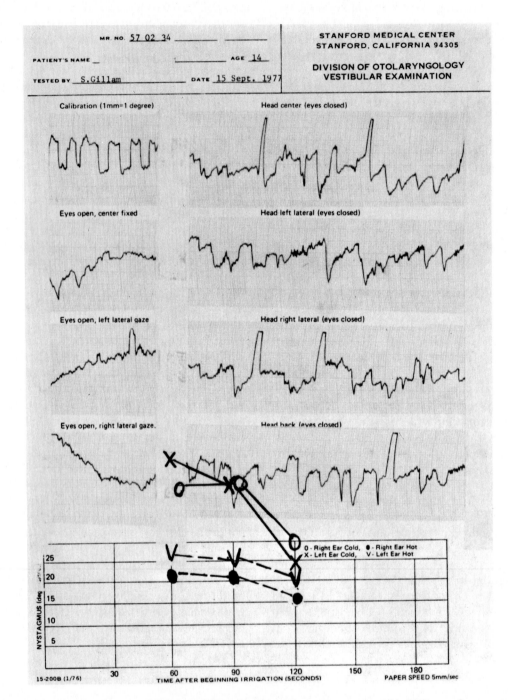

Figs. 3-2 and 3-3. Mounted segments of the ENG which accompany the written report. This ENG was chosen as an illustration because two of the three abnormalities described are fairly common and strongly suggest that this patient was hyperaroused or "nervous" during the test. Accentuated random saccades are seen throughout the positional testing, and in the mounted segments of the figure the head-back position is a good illustration. Quite often, this sign of emotional tension is accompanied by a second sign, hyperactive responses to calorics. While such bilateral hyperactivity can be caused by a very rare midline cerebellar lesion, it more commonly reflects the patient's emotional state.

22

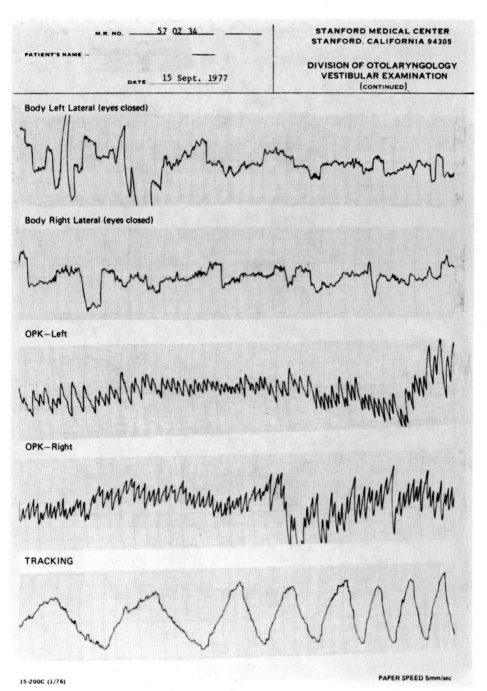

Body Left Lateral (eyes closed)

Body Right Lateral (eyes closed)

OPK—Left

OPK—Right

TRACKING

15-200C (1/76)

PAPER SPEED 5mm/sec

Fig. 3-3.

MEDICAL RECORD NO. 57 02 34

PATIENT'S NAME __

DATE: 15 Sept. 1977 AGE: 14

STANFORD MEDICAL CENTER
STANFORD, CALIFORNIA 94305

DIVISION OF OTOLARYNGOLOGY
VESTIBULAR EXAMINATION
REPORT

There is no gaze or position-induced nystagmus. A left-beating spontaneous nystagmus is present at the approximate rate of 5-8°/sec. This nystagmus is decreased with the head turned to the right and maybe with the body rotated to the right. Optokinetic nystagmus is symmetrical. There is an increase in saccades and muscle tremor.

Bithermal caloric-induced nystagmus is symmetrical but the responses are hyperactive.

Impression: Abnormal examination.
1. spontaneous nystagmus
2. increased saccades and muscle tremor
3. hyperactive caloric responses

M.D.

Fig. 3-4. Final written report generated from the work sheet.

4.

THE ENG WHOLEMOUNTS

The ENG wholemounts in this atlas are not completely typical of the average day-to-day ENGs. There are very few borderline examinations. They do contain at least one example of almost every abnormality that one is likely to encounter in several years of ENG experience. They also include some deliberate mistakes, artifacts, and other problems you can also expect to encounter. Part of any ENG interpretation is detecting fact from artifact and significant from insignificant.

The principal merit of these tracings is their entirety—the complete unedited ENG tracing. Study each one and take notes on the abnormalities. Plot the caloric-induced nystagmus velocities. Then, and only then, read the text. In other words, use the atlas as if it were a programmed instruction guide. Remember that the case histories of these ENG patients were collected *after* we decided that the ENG was to be included in this atlas, not the reverse. Had we used the case histories to select the ENGs, the sample would probably have been much different. The case histories and physical findings are accurate. Most negative clinical findings have been omitted for brevity.

Some tracings have both horizontal and vertical eye-motion tracings. There is no special reason for the vertical leads except that the tracings were obtained during a period of almost 3 years when we recorded all ENGs this way. We no longer do this routinely because the amount of additional information obtained did not justify the effort. Read at least a few of these, especially those in which there is a nystagmus vector present.

WHOLEMOUNT LAYOUT AND LABELING

Refer to ENG-1 as an example. Each tracing reads from left to right. The several lines of strip-chart paper are sequential, usually without any editing. In some long ENGs (typically those with additional calorics), segments have been abbreviated, and these will be obvious.

Magnification will make reading easier. The wholemount can be enlarged by using an opaque projector or a magnifying glass.

All labeling (eyes-center, eyes-closed, head-left, etc.) is placed directly above the beginning of that segment of the test. Labeling appears below the vertical tracings. The optokinetic and pursuit-tracking tests, when present, are not always labeled in great detail. When the OPN responses appear to be abnormal, there will usually be two drum speeds, and the transitions from one speed to another are usually not labeled. Pursuit trackings are of two types: pendular—characterized in the normal but nearly perfect sine waves on the strip chart, usually at two (sometimes three) speeds; and sawtooth— slow, even movement of the light stimulus to the left or right with an instantaneous return to the starting point, also at two or three speeds. Normal responses should look like a sawtooth ramp on the strip chart. A three-speed pendular tracking, but not ramp tracking, is shown on ENG-1.

A second calibration section is done just before the OPN test or just after the last positioning test and an unlabeled segment of this calibration is mounted on the right-hand side of the wholemount, just above the caloric responses. All calibrations are at 10 mm of pen deflection for 10° of visual arc displacement. The photo reduction from the original trace is at a ratio of about 3.3:1. During some caloric nystagmus the amplification is reduced by one-half when the velocity is extremely rapid. These segments are labeled "½ calibration." Eye movements of possible clinical significance are visible without magnification in most instances, however. Those that cannot be easily seen have been enlarged and reproduced as figures.

Paper speed is 5 mm/sec, and this corresponds to about 1.5 cm per each 10 seconds on the photo reduction. A 25 mm/sec paper speed is used occasionally to define eye movements more closely. These segments are identified.

The slow-phase velocity scale at the lower right of ENG-1 can be used to calculate slow-phase velocity directly off the wholemounts. The size reduction is likely to lead to errors, however, so some magnification would be helpful. With or without magnification, the best way to proceed is to draw a straight line along the slow-phase vector of several nystagmus beats that occur within, say, 10 seconds. Then use the average line slope to match against the scale. It is much more accurate to use the visually determined average slope of several beats because the slow-phase velocity can vary from beat to beat. For an example, see the final seconds of the right warm caloric. Slope A seems about average.

For better accuracy in calculating the slow-phase velocity, use the calibrations immediately after each caloric. The first few trackings of these calibrations have not been readjusted to yield 10 mm of pen deflection and will thus reflect the actual eye speed during the caloric nystagmus. Sometimes it is important to adjust the estimates of slow-phase velocity using these calibrations. Large changes in the skin-electrode resistance do occur during caloric stimulations. These changes affect the calibration and can lead to false velocity values. For example, suppose that the 10° calibration has become 15 mm after a caloric and that the calculated slow-phase velocity, using the scale calibrated for 10°, is 25° per second at 90 seconds. The true velocity is more likely ten-fifteenths or two-thirds of 25° per second. (See ENG-37, for example.)

The symbols used for the caloric-induced nystagmus velocities are shown in Figure 4-1.

MEASURED
WITH EYES OPEN

RIGHT COLD	O	OO
LEFT COLD	X	XX
RIGHT HOT	●	●●
LEFT HOT	V	V V
RIGHT ICE	△	△△
LEFT ICE	▯	▯▯

Fig. 4-1. Symbols used in plotting the slow phase of caloric-induced nystagmus.

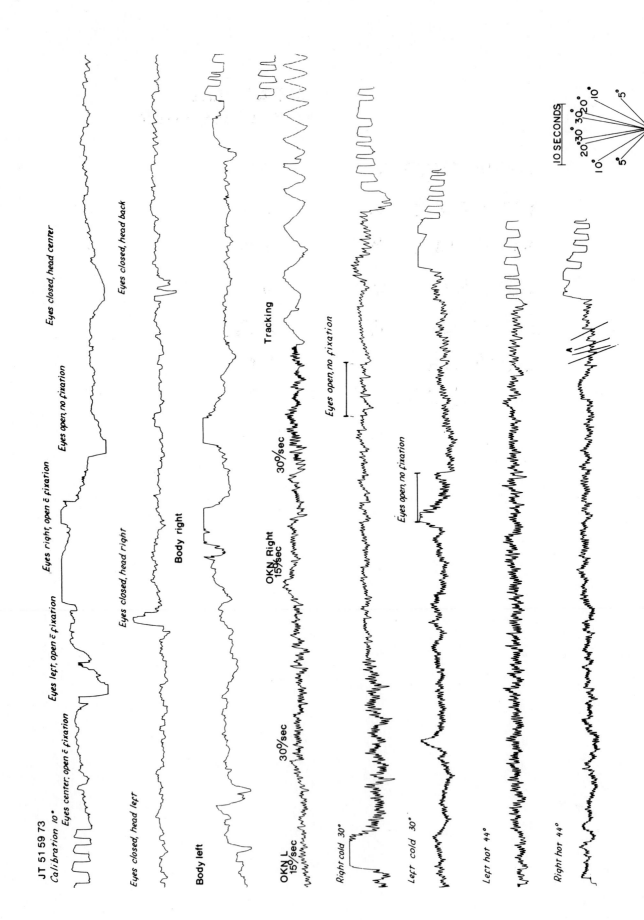

ENG-1.

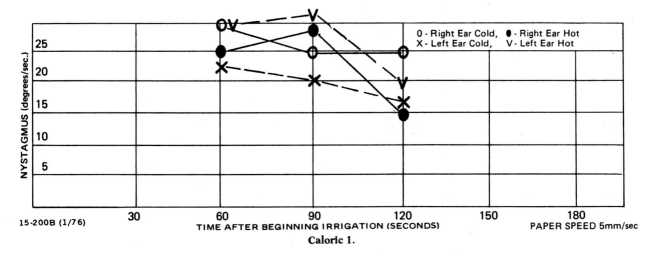

15-200B (1/76)

TIME AFTER BEGINNING IRRIGATION (SECONDS)

PAPER SPEED 5mm/sec

Caloric 1.

ENG-1

History: A 72-year-old female complains of intermittent left facial pain and dizziness of 6 months' duration. She is quite vague about her dizziness, but it seems to be a light-headedness which is worse in the morning. She has no focal neurological symptoms. An audiogram shows a sloping, bilateral, high-frequency sensorineural hearing loss, worse on the left, and good discrimination bilaterally. She has a history of recurrent rhinosinusitis. Examination and neurological tests are normal except for mild tenderness localized in the left temporomandibular joint.

ENG Report: There is no gaze, spontaneous, or position-induced nystagmus. Optokinetic nystagmus is symmetrical.

Bithermal caloric-induced nystagmus is within normal limits for nystagmus velocity and right-left symmetry.

IMPRESSION. Normal examination.

Comment: This is a remarkably good tracing for a 72-year-old person. There are a few beats of left nystagmus immediately after the head-right positioning, which are well within normal limits. The caloric nystagmus indicates a high level of arousal in which the patient keeps her eyes near the midplane by short saccades at frequent intervals. In general, small-amplitude caloric nystagmus indicates good arousal, whereas irregular large amplitude waveforms can suggest poor arousal.

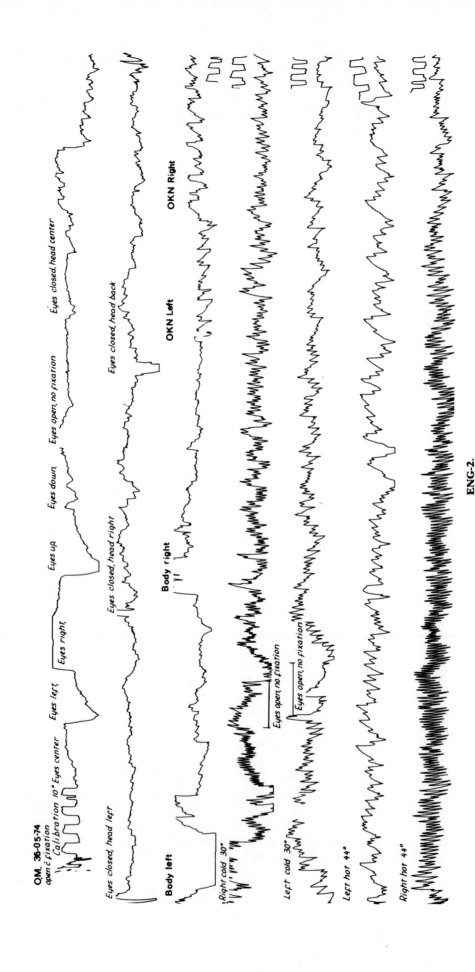

ENG-2.

30

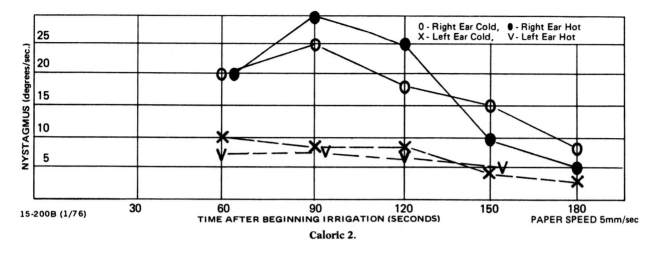

Caloric 2.

ENG-2

History: This 52-year-old female has a 10-year history of intermittent dizziness, nausea and vomiting, tinnitus, and decreased hearing in her left ear. Her audiogram shows a flat 70-dB sensorineural loss on the left, 30 percent speech discrimination, complete recruitment, no tone decay, and a Type II Békésy tracing. Neurological examination is normal.

ENG Report: There is no gaze or fixation nystagmus. There is an irregularly present left-beating spontaneous nystagmus (approximate velocity 3°–5° per second) which changes to a slight right-beating nystagmus in the head- and body-left positions. OPN is poorly executed but probably normal.
Caloric-induced nystagmus is hypoactive on the left.

IMPRESSION. Abnormal examination, spontaneous nystagmus with a position-induced, direction-changing component, and hypoactive left calorics.

Diagnosis: Meniere's syndrome.

Comment: The spontaneous nystagmus here is not very impressive and neither is its direction reversal and does not merit much clinical attention. The depressed calorics are consistent with this woman's 10-year history of Meniere's attacks. Most individuals with very recent onsets of Meniere's syndrome do not have consistently depressed calorics but have fluctuations similar to their hearing. Also, long-standing damage to the end-organ is typically coupled with less spontaneous nystagmus than are recent damages.

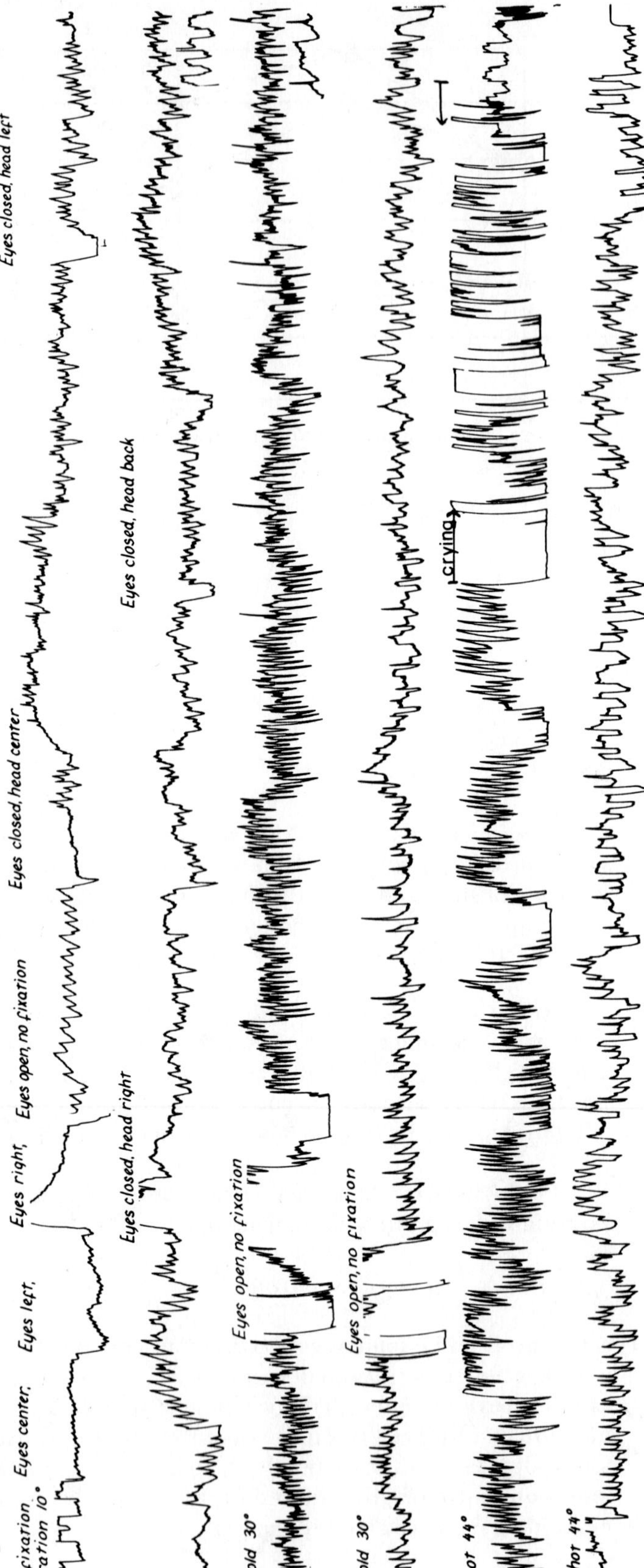

DN 27 44 79

open c̄ fixation. Eyes center, Eyes left, Eyes right, Eyes open, no fixation Eyes closed, head center Eyes closed, head left

Calibration 10°

Eyes closed, head right

Right cold 30° Eyes open, no fixation Eyes closed, head back

Left cold 30° Eyes open, no fixation

Left hot 44° crying

Right hot 44°

ENG-3.

32

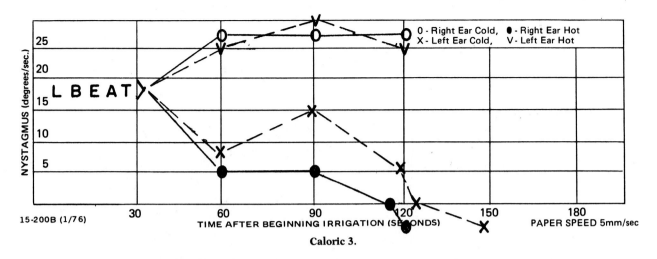

Caloric 3.

ENG-3

History: A 48-year-old female has noticed for the past several months that turning her head to the left induced a definite spatial disorientation. About 6 days ago, she had the sudden onset of severe and persistent vertigo with the sensation that objects were jerking from left to right. This occurs somewhat more prominently when she turns her eyes to the left rather than to the right. Recently, she has developed unsteadiness of gait, with a tendency to fall to the left. She does not have diplopia, dysarthria, dysphagia, limb weakness, or paresthesia. She probably had an episode of retrobulbar neuritis 2½ years ago.

On exam, there is optic atrophy in the left eye and moderately decreased vision. There is rotary nystagmus to the left which is increased on left gaze. The patient is unable to perform tandem walking. Neurological exam is otherwise normal. She has slightly decreased hearing on the right.

ENG Report: There is no gaze nystagmus. There is a spontaneous, left-beating nystagmus with an average velocity of about 10° per second with the eyes open and vision fixed. This velocity remains about the same with fixation prevented (amplitude increases as expected), but with lids closed, the nystagmus increases to 15°–20° per second (again, as expected). This spontaneous nystagmus is moderately inhibited by visual fixation to the right (see calibration tracking or gaze tests) and is moderately inhibited in the head-right position.

Bithermal caloric-induced nystagmus is abnormal and difficult to interpret because of the marked spontaneous nystagmus. It is, for example, difficult to determine the exact velocity of the response to right-cool stimulation because of the superimposed vectors of both to the left. Caloric responses are those of a nystagmus preponderance to the left, probably as a result of this.

IMPRESSION. Abnormal exam, spontaneous nystagmus that is affected by head position, and caloric-induced nystagmus preponderance to the left.

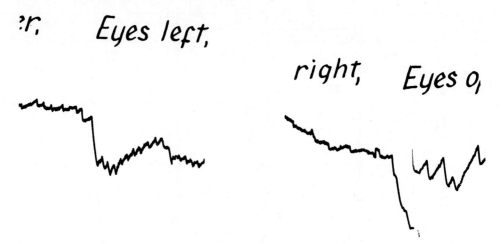

Fig. ENG-3-1. (A) Eyes center going to eyes left. (B) Eyes right going to eyes open without fixation.

NOTE.   This exam should be repeated in about 3 weeks for comparison with today's ENG. Her clinical history suggests a *peripheral labyrinthine defect* (now acute), and depending upon how this resolves in a few weeks, it will be a bit easier to detect which ear is involved.

Diagnosis: Peripheral labyrinthine disease versus central demyelinating disease (multiple sclerosis).

Follow-up: The patient has had further evidence of demyelinating disease and has been treated with ACTH.

Comment: The "gaze" nystagmus in this ENG (see Fig. ENG-3-1) is not a pathological gaze nystagmus but an accentuated vestibular nystagmus upon gaze in the direction of the fast component. Alexander's law states that the spontaneous nystagmus associated with an acute peripheral vestibular lesion beats strongest on gaze in the direction of the quick component, less in the primary position, and least in the direction of the slow component. This is sometimes called first-, second-, and third-degree spontaneous nystagmus.[1] This example is clear-cut, since the spontaneous nystagmus obeys all the rules for peripheral vestibular origin—increasing amplitude and velocity as visual inhibition is increased, first by preventing fixation and then by lid closure, and finally suppression (or enhancement) with head positioning.

It is sometimes difficult to know if a unidirectional "gaze" nystagmus is pathological when a less-impressive spontaneous nystagmus is also present but observed only with the eyes closed. It is probably best in such instances to reserve judgment about a "gaze" abnormality's clinical importance.

There is also considerable eye blinking during the caloric stimulations, especially when the fast phase of the nystagmus is to the right. Here, as in most blink artifacts, the direction of the pen deflection remains constant (upwards here) throughout the ENG. (See ENG-4.)

Contrary to what is sometimes said in the literature, there is no specific ENG pattern for multiple sclerosis.

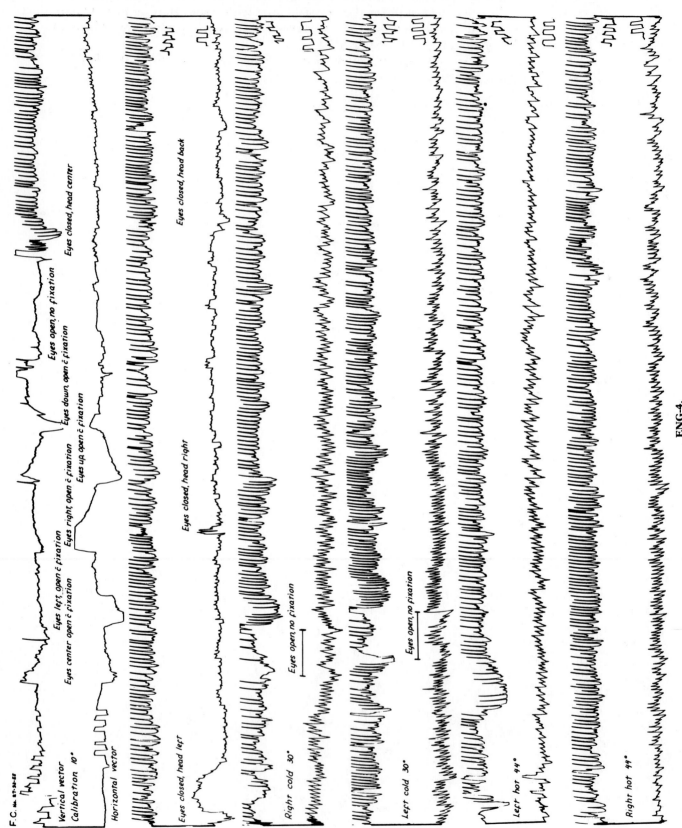

F.C. No. 87-22-25

Vertical vector
Calibration 10°

Horizontal vector

Eyes center open c̄ fixation

Eyes left, open c̄ fixation

Eyes right, open c̄ fixation

Eyes down, open c̄ fixation

Eyes up open c̄ fixation

Eyes open, no fixation

Eyes open c̄ fixation

Eyes closed, head center

Eyes closed, head left

Eyes closed, head back

Eyes closed, head right

Right cold 30°

Eyes open, no fixation

Left cold 30°

Eyes open, no fixation

Left hot 44°

Right hot 44°

ENG-4.

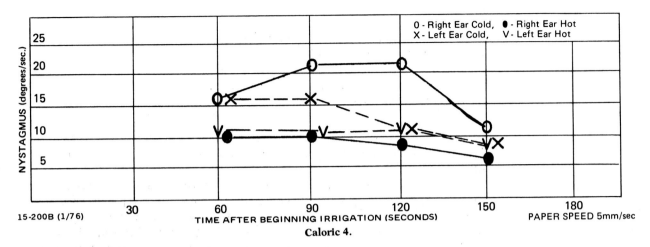

Caloric 4.

15-200B (1/76)   TIME AFTER BEGINNING IRRIGATION (SECONDS)   PAPER SPEED 5mm/sec

ENG-4

History: A 53-year-old female presents with 1½ years of intermittent dizziness beginning with the sudden onset of a left hemiparesis. Arteriograms were reported as normal, and she was placed on antihypertensive therapy. In the past month, she reports two episodes of loss of balance in the upright position associated with tinnitus of short duration. She has no other neurological symptoms. Examination shows a slight droop of the left corner of the mouth and a mild weakness in both left extremities. There is a mild right sensorineural hearing loss with good discrimination, negative tone decay, and no recruitment. Metabolic workup is negative.

ENG Report: There is a physiological gaze nystagmus during left lateral gaze. There may be a slight left-beating spontaneous nystagmus, but eye-blink artifact is more likely.

Bithermal caloric-induced nystagmus is within normal limits for nystagmus velocity and right-left symmetry.

IMPRESSION. Normal examination.

Working Diagnosis: Possible basilar artery insufficiency versus possible Meniere's syndrome.

Comment: The vertical tracing with eyes closed shows a rhythmic eye-blink artifact. This can also be seen in horizontal tracings (Fig. ENG-4-1). Eye-blink artifact is usually easy to detect, but not always, especially if the reader is not familiar with tracings from a particular ENG machine.

Most clinical ENG machines have an alternating current (AC) time constant that serves as a low-frequency filter. The effect is to cause a steady-state or tonic eye deviation to appear as if it is slowly returning to the midline at a rate equal to the low-frequency time constant of the machine (Fig. ENG-4-2A). The clearest normal example of this is seen during "gaze" testing.

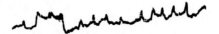

Fig. 4-1. Symbols used in plotting the slow phase of caloric-induced nystagmus.

A nystagmus beat's velocity exceeds the time constant of the recorder, and thus the slope reflects the rate of eye movement with reasonable accuracy (Fig. ENG-4-2C).

A high-frequency event, such as an eye blink, appears as a typical spike pattern. The very end of a blink, however, returns to baseline at a rate dependent upon the time constant of the machine. This part of the blink can be mistaken for nystagmus, especially when blinking is rhythmic (Fig. ENG-4-2B). There may be considerable variability between machines in both time constant and high-frequency response which may alter the shape of eye-blink tracings.[40] In fact, some machines with exceptionally poor high-frequency response do not record the blink spike. Thus, distinguishing blink from nystagmus is nearly impossible. If you are unfam-

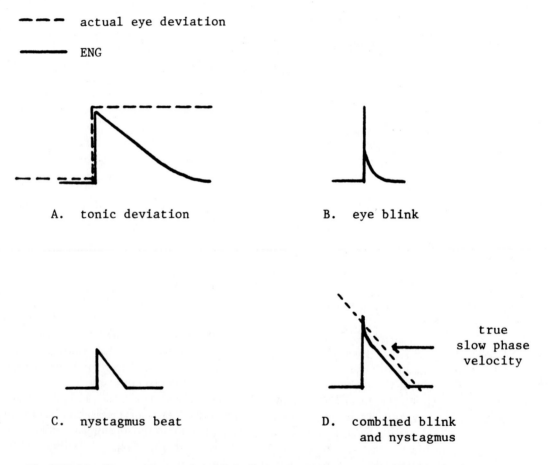

Fig. ENG-4-2. Time constant and eye blink effect on an AC ENG recording. See text for descriptions.

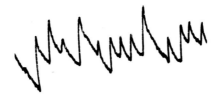

Fig. ENG-4-3. Segment of left-cool caloric at about 2.5 minutes.

iliar with an ENG machine's tracings, or suspect yours has a poor high-frequency response, look elsewhere on the tracing for evidence. A good indicator is the OPN tracing. The peaks between the fast and slow phases should be sharp, not rounded.

The most complex situation occurs when blinks are synchronous with nystagmus beats as seen on this ENG (Fig. ENG-4-3). The nystagmus appears to have a sharp spike superimposed upon the fast phase. When the slow-phase velocity is calculated, the upper peaked part of the tracing must be ignored and only the slow-phase velocity used. (Fig. ENG-4-2D)

Follow-up: Eight years later, the patient has infrequent dizzy spells and no change in her hearing. She requires mild antihypertensive therapy.

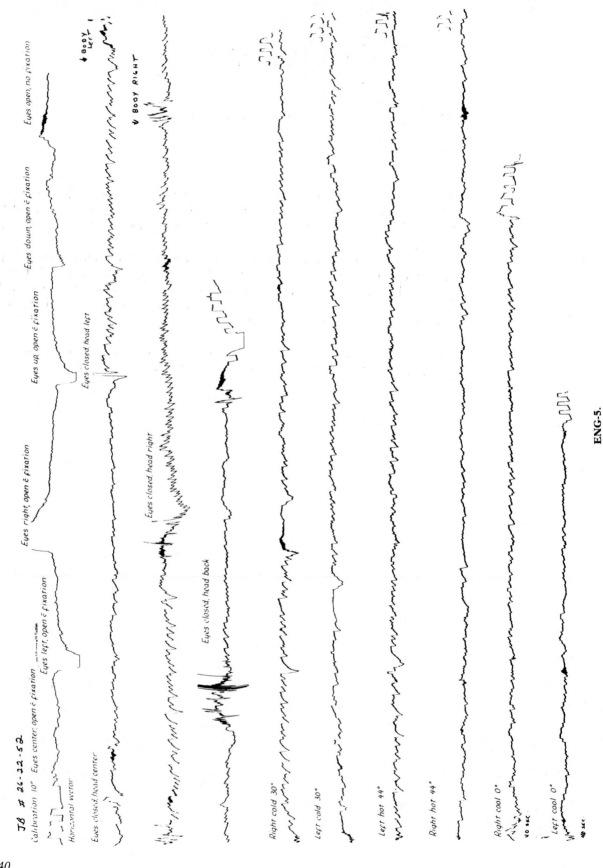

40

ENG-5.

ENG-5

History: A 44-year-old female presents with a 2-year history of "drop attacks" in which she suddenly loses her balance and collapses without any associated nausea or true vertigo. There is no associated disturbance of consciousness, and she recognizes no precipitating cause or symptom. Twenty years ago, she had an episode of blindness in one eye lasting 1 hour. This symptom has never recurred. There are no other focal neurological symptoms. She has taken diazepam and diamphetamine in the past.

EEGs and cerebral arteriogram are normal, and a pneumoencephalogram shows "mild dilation of the lateral ventricles." Audiometry is normal. Examination shows questionable left gaze nystagmus and slight ataxia on tandem gait.

ENG Report: There is no gaze nystagmus. There is a slight left-beating spontaneous nystagmus with eyes closed (average velocity approximately 1°–3° per second). There is a marked direction-changing, position-induced nystagmus in the lateral head positions (average velocity to the left, 10° per second; to the right, 8°–10° per second). There was no appreciable change in the nystagmus when neck torsion was avoided by rotating her body to the right and left.

There is no response to bithermal caloric tests nor to maximum stimulus of 5 ml of ice water in either ear.

IMPRESSION.   Abnormal examination; spontaneous left-beating nystagmus; direction-changing, position-induced nystagmus; no response to calorics.

Differential Diagnosis: Includes multiple sclerosis and early posterior fossa tumor by the neurology department.

Long-term Follow-up: Follow-up of the patient 8 years later found her asymptomatic on small doses of antiepileptic drugs.

Comment: The most striking finding here is the complete loss of caloric nystagmus in a patient with minimal historic physical findings. In such a patient with normal hearing, the principal causes have been midline posterior fossa tumors, autoimmune syndromes, ototoxic drugs, and congenital disease. About 12 percent of cases remain unknown.[39] The reason for this patient's loss of caloric nystagmus falls in the latter category. It is possible that some slight response to caloric testing does exist here if one pays tribute to the slight increment in the right-cool and left-warm stimulus responses while ignoring the ice water stimulations. The stronger stimuli seem to have less effect. This is very unlikely. Instead, I strongly suspect that whatever "response" seems present to the bithermal calorics is caused by increased patient arousal and thereby an increase in the background spontaneous nystagmus. (See ENG-9, 30, and 34 for other examples and comments.)

Her "spontaneous nystagmus" is minor compared with the position-induced, direction-changing nystagmus. This positional nystagmus is not related to the caloric findings. Persons with nonresponsive calorics typically have fairly random eyes-closed eye motions. Here, the likely cause is evenly split between sedative drugs and an unknown CNS debility. Eight years of asymptomatic survival strongly suggest drugs. A repeat ENG or sedative-drug blood levels would have helped in deciding between these two.

The "body-right" and "body-left" positional tests were performed on the slight chance that the positional nystagmus might have been caused by neck torsion rather than by head position. Turning the patient's body left and right, without rotating the neck, may eliminate such effects and could thus be theoretically helpful in localizing cause (but also see the Comments section of ENG-27).

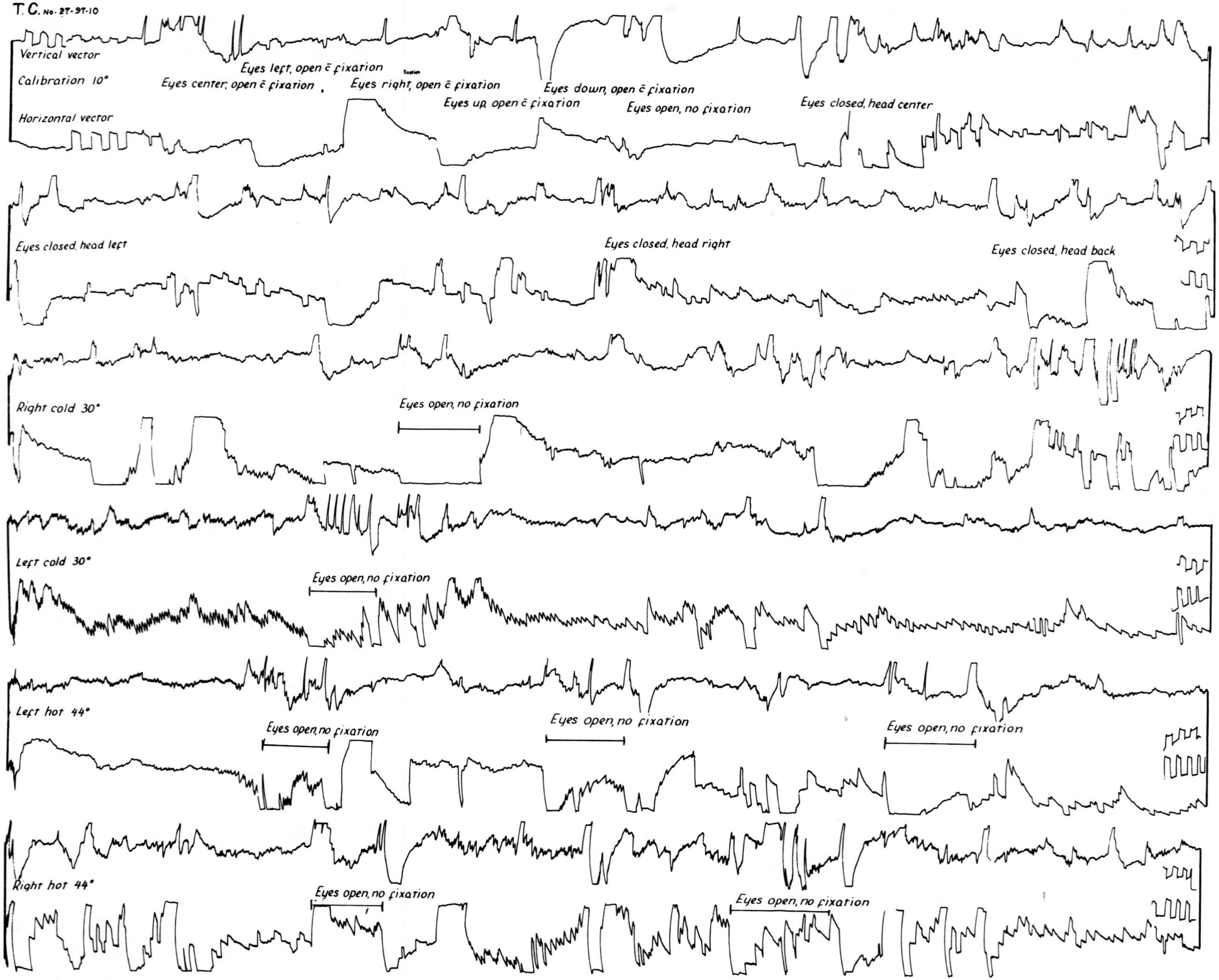

T.C. No. 27-57-10

Vertical vector

Calibration 10°

Horizontal vector

Eyes center, open c̄ fixation

Eyes left, open c̄ fixation fixation

Eyes right, open c̄ fixation .

Eyes down, open c̄ fixation

Eyes open, no fixation

Eyes closed, head center

Eyes closed, head back

Eyes up, open c̄ fixation

Eyes closed, head left

Eyes closed, head right

Right cold 30°

Eyes open, no fixation

Left cold 30°

Eyes open, no fixation

Left hot 44°

Eyes open, no fixation

Eyes open, no fixation

Eyes open, no fixation

Right hot 44°

Eyes open, no fixation

Eyes open, no fixation

ENG-6.

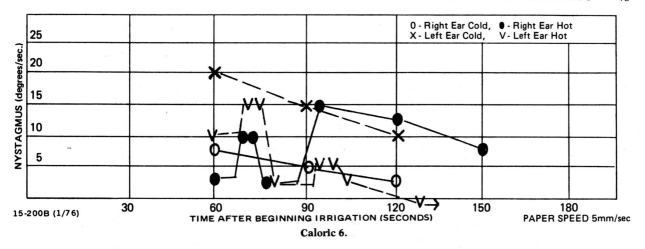

Caloric 6.

15-200B (1/76)   TIME AFTER BEGINNING IRRIGATION (SECONDS)   PAPER SPEED 5mm/sec

0 - Right Ear Cold,   ● - Right Ear Hot
X - Left Ear Cold,   V - Left Ear Hot

ENG-6

History: A 41-year-old female has increasingly severe intermittent imbalance for 2 years. The episodes have a spontaneous onset and last for seconds to minutes. She has no true vertigo, but she does have the feeling of passing out or falling. Her history includes recurrent left serous otitis media and a myringotomy 2 years ago. She has a mild right sensorineural hearing loss and a left 15-dB conductive hearing loss. Examination and workup are normal, including brain scan, EEG, and lumbar puncture.

ENG Report: There is a physiological left gaze nystagmus and a very low-grade, intermittent right-beating spontaneous nystagmus that is increased in the head-right and probably in the head-back positions.

The caloric stimulations are not totally technically satisfactory. There may be a loose electrode causing intermittent wide swings in the pen tracing. The right-cool response is definitely hypoactive. If a loose electrode can be excluded, there is a tonic deviation of the eyes to the left, which may account for the intermittent nature of the response to the right-cool caloric. This test should be repeated if clinically indicated, at no charge to the patient.

IMPRESSION. Abnormal ENG because of a low-grade spontaneous nystagmus that is affected by head position; abnormal calorics that may contain technical artifacts.

Diagnosis: None. The patient has been treated successfully with tranquilizers.

Comment: The differential diagnosis of artifacts versus real findings in an ENG can be a difficult problem. In general, it is best to repeat the test rather than guess. Note the pen swings to the left when the eyes are opened during calorics. This could represent tonic eye deviation to the right while the eyes are closed. This response is inconsistent, however, and the multiple, apparently random wide swings in the tracing are probably the result of a loose electrode. Suspect an electrode problem when there are wide swings onto the baseline at those times during the test when the patient moves. Note here that major deflections occurred when the eyes were closed or when the head position changed.

There is also some suggestion that the patient's level of arousal was not optimal. See, for example, the variations in nystagmus following the right-cool irrigation.

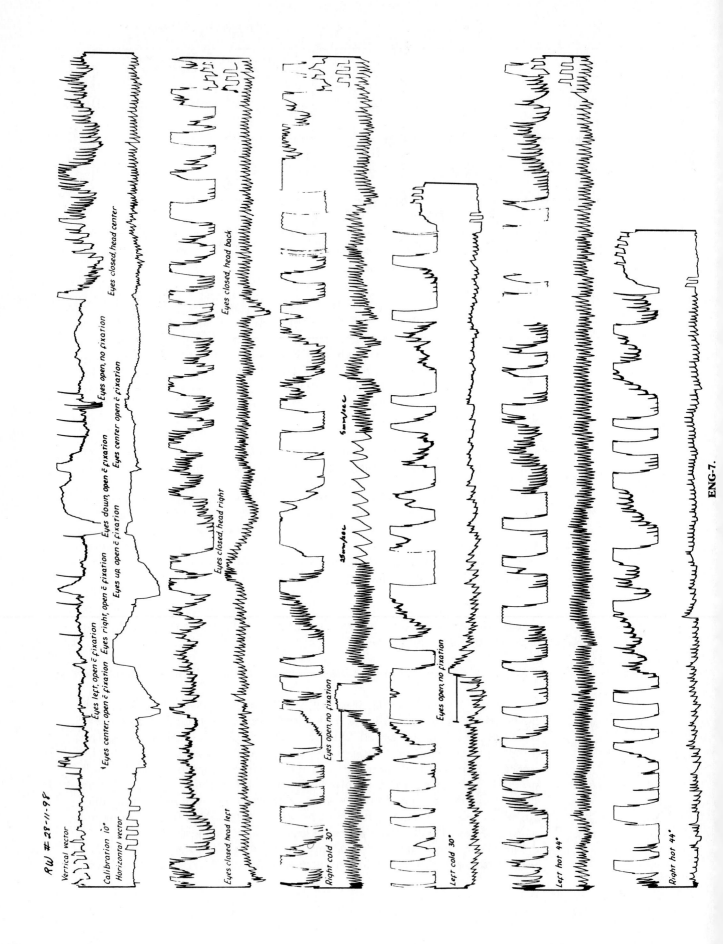

ENG-7.

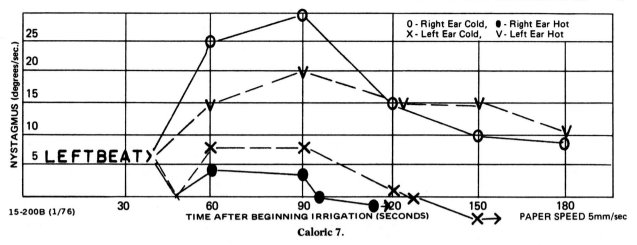

Caloric 7.

15-200B (1/76)

TIME AFTER BEGINNING IRRIGATION (SECONDS)   PAPER SPEED 5mm/sec

ENG-7

History: A 43-year-old male is referred with a 3-month history of frequent (two to three per week) episodes of vertigo, feeling of fullness, and decreased hearing in the left ear. He has been treated with antihistamines and a low-sodium diet without relief. Examination is normal. There is a moderate sensorineural hearing loss on the left, with a speech reception threshold (SRT) of 50 dB, 88 percent discrimination, positive short-increment sensitivity index (SISI), and complete recruitment.

ENG Report: There is no gaze nystagmus. There is a left-beating spontaneous nystagmus both with the eyes open (slight) and with the eyes closed (approximate rate 7°–10° per second). This spontaneous nystagmus is slightly increased in the head-right position. There is a marked increased in eye blinks when the eyes are closed.

Bithermal caloric-induced nystagmus is asymmetrical, demonstrating a left directional preponderance. This preponderance probably was caused by the superimposition of the above-mentioned spontaneous nystagmus vector, probably with normal caloric responses underneath.

IMPRESSION.   Abnormal examination, spontaneous nystagmus, directional preponderance to the left.

Diagnosis: Probable Meniere's syndrome, but the patient said his symptoms improved after getting his "neck stretched" by a chiropractor.

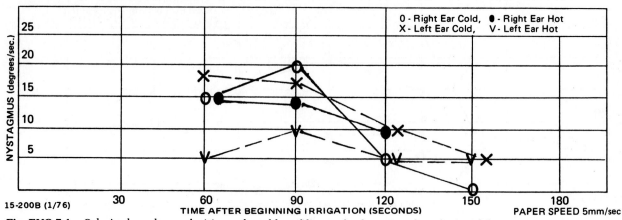

Fig. ENG-7-1. Caloric slow-phase velocities replotted by adding and subtracting the velocity of the spontaneous nystagmus.

Follow-up: Seven years later the patient is asymptomatic and still insists he was cured by the chiropractor.

Comment: This patient was retested 1½ years later, and the results showed a marked change toward normal; only position-induced nystagmus was present, and the calorics were normal.

In evaluating directional preponderance, it must be remembered that this is a nonspecific response and may be either central or peripheral in origin. In fact, the directional preponderance exhibited by this patient was probably due to the underlying spontaneous nystagmus. Figure ENG-7-1 shows the caloric responses "corrected" for a possible spontaneous nystagmus influence.

There are no clear rules for deciding when a spontaneous nystagmus is interacting with the caloric nystagmus. Some interpreters use such corrections routinely when a spontaneous nystagmus is present. I do not, mainly because such corrections can lead to as many interpretive errors as they appear to solve. Suppose, for example, that a spontaneous nystagmus is present and the caloric nystagmus is normal and symmetrical. Adding and subtracting vectors would create a nystagmus preponderance. Thus, while there is sometimes a relation between calorics and spontaneous nystagmus, more investigative work is needed before rules are applied.

In this instance, the caloric tests are of no help in substantiating which ear (if either) was involved in this patient's dizziness problem. If the issue of right or left ear becomes important in clinical management and this cannot be substantiated by other means (such as an audiogram), repeat caloric testing at 2- to 3-week intervals is sometimes quite helpful. Caloric responses can fluctuate in much the same manner as do audiograms in Meniere's patients.

There is also a considerable amount of blink artifact present in this record (see vertical vector tracings), and this blinking is more prominent in certain head positions than in other head positions. In this instance, the blink is synchronized with the onset of the fast phase of the nystagmus. This is the normal and the expected pattern. In calculating slow-phase velocities, however, it is important to omit the blink artifact by calculating only the easily measurable portions of the slow phase and not the "peaked tips." (See ENG-4.)

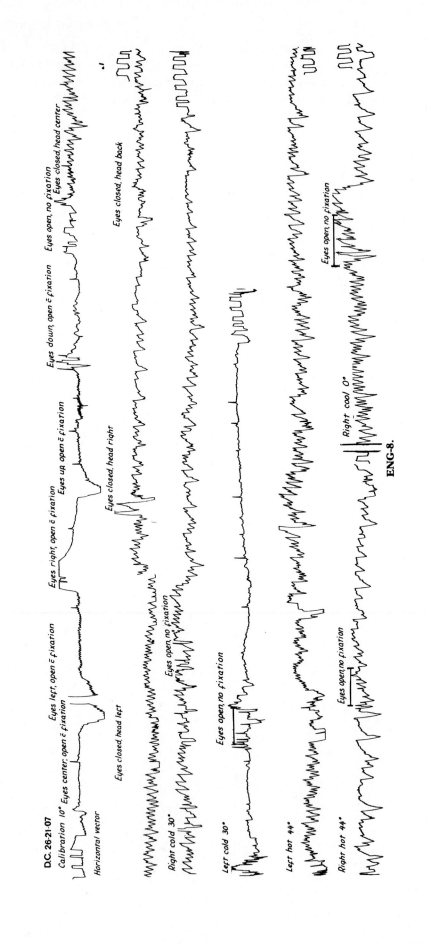

ENG-8.

50

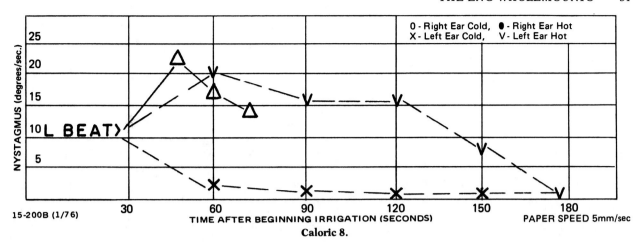

Caloric 8.

15-200B (1/76)

TIME AFTER BEGINNING IRRIGATION (SECONDS)

PAPER SPEED 5mm/sec

NYSTAGMUS (degrees/sec.)

0 - Right Ear Cold, ● - Right Ear Hot
X - Left Ear Cold, V - Left Ear Hot

L BEAT

ENG-8

History: A 60-year-old male has had three episodes of severe vertigo in the past 12 years that were associated with nausea and vomiting and are aggravated by position. He has never had fluctuation of his hearing. The most recent attack began 1 week ago. He had a slightly decreased right corneal reflex and a slight tendency to fall to the right during tandem walking. There was a bilateral sensorineural hearing loss with recruitment, normal discrimination, and negative tone decay. He was mildly hypertensive. Workup showed an abnormal glucose tolerance test and elevated triglycerides and cholesterol. He had grade II atherosclerotic changes in his fundi, peripheral vascular insufficiency in his legs, but no neck bruits. EEG was normal.

ENG Report: There is a very fine and regular left-gaze nystagmus which is probably not a true visual event but rather a reflection of the left-beating spontaneous nystagmus that is seen in the eyes-closed position. The distinction between a true gaze nystagmus and a vestibular nystagmus that is accentuated by eye position is difficult from this tracing, mainly because the strip recording of the eyes center, open, without fixation is too short and technically poor. One would normally also expect to see a vestibular-induced nystagmus in this position.

The spontaneous nystagmus that is clearly present has an average velocity of 10° per second in the head-center position. It is suppressed to an average velocity of 3° per second in the head-right position.

Bithermal caloric-induced nystagmus is abnormal. There is no appreciable decrement or increment to the left-beating spontaneous nystagmus during the right ear stimulations. There are responses from the left ear that have a significant effect on the superimposed spontaneous nystagmus. There is probably a response present to stimulation of the right ear with ice water.

IMPRESSION. Abnormal examination, spontaneous nystagmus that is affected by head position, probably severely hypoactive right-ear calorics.

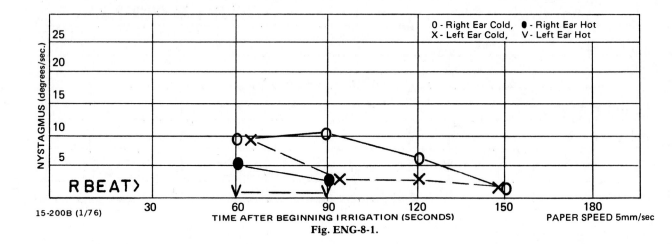

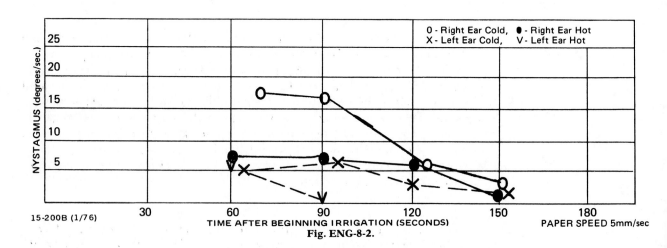

Fig. ENG-8-1.

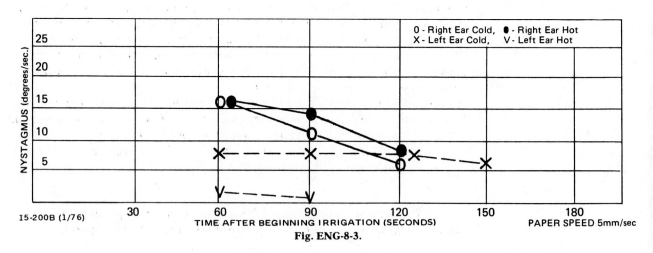

Fig. ENG-8-2.

Fig. ENG-8-3.

Figs. ENG-8-1,2, and 3. Serial calorics obtained at approximately 2-week intervals after the first ENG.

52

Diagnosis: Acute labyrinthine upset.

Follow-up: Patient improved in the hospital on rest, Dramamine, and Antivert. Follow-up 1 year later shows no change in symptoms and no evidence of basilar artery disease.

To delineate this problem further, serial ENGs were performed at approximately weekly intervals.

EXAM NUMBER 2.   There was a spontaneous right-beating nystagmus when the eyes were closed (direction reversed from previous exam). Caloric responses now show only modest depressions to the right ear stimuli, and no response to the left-warm irrigation (see Fig. ENG-8-1). This failure to arouse a left-warm stimulation may have been due to the superimposition of the right-beating spontaneous nystagmus, but there is no way to determine this with certainty.

EXAM NUMBER 3.   The spontaneous nystagmus has disappeared completely. There is no head position effect. Caloric responses remain about the same as in exam number 2 (see Fig. ENG-8-2).

EXAM NUMBER 4.   There is neither gaze nystagmus nor spontaneous nystagmus. There is a transient right-beating nystagmus for the first 30 seconds after turning the head to the left. Bithermal caloric-induced nystagmus shows a definite left hypoactivity (see Fig. ENG-8-3).

Comment: Serial ENGs were obtained on this patient because of a differential diagnostic problem—brain stem ischemia versus Meniere's syndrome.

This serial set of ENGs emphasizes that during an acute episode of vertigo, findings may be quite different than when the patient is relatively asymptomatic. Thus, it is valuable to consider repeat testing when the sidedness, or even the location, of an abnormality is in doubt. Specific points from this case are as follows: (1) the direction of a spontaneous nystagmus is not a reliable index of which ear is involved; (2) caloric irrigations do not always specify which ear is producing symptoms. Involvement here may in fact have been bilateral.

Serial caloric irrigations at 1- to 2-week intervals can also be useful in detecting which ear is responsible for symptoms of Meniere's syndrome when the initial examination for hearing and vestibular function is symmetrical. Vestibular function, like hearing, often fluctuates.

ENG-9.

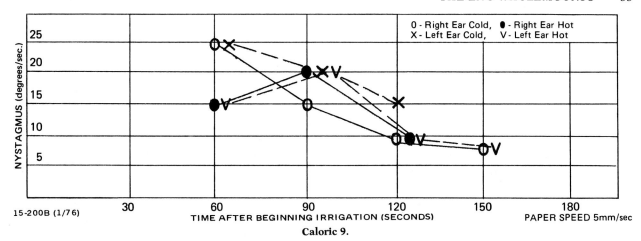

Caloric 9.

15-200B (1/76)

ENG-9

History: A 44-year-old female complains of headaches and vertigo since an auto accident 1 year ago. She suffered muscle strain in the right neck and shoulder, but probably no head injury and no loss of consciousness. She feels a lightness in the head, things get black, and she must hold onto something. She has "passed out" once and has fallen several times. Her attacks are unpredictable, and she has had them in bed. She also complains of an inability to concentrate. Physical and neurological examination is normal. The audiogram is normal.

ONE EXAMINER'S COMMENT. "Patient appears to be 'out of it'—in a world of her own but quite cooperative in spite of it."

ENG Report: There is no gaze, spontaneous, or position-induced nystagmus present with eyes open or closed.

Bithermal caloric-induced nystagmus is within normal limits for nystagmus velocity and right-left symmetry.

There is considerable irregularity in the baseline of this tracing during both steady-state and caloric tests. Most of this is the result of random eye motion and probably a general nervousness during testing.

IMPRESSION. Normal examination.

Clinical Impression: Psychosomatic spatial disorientation disorder.

Comment: An increase in random saccades is almost always an indication of anxiety or a highly aroused patient. Sometimes this suggestion of anxiety is clinically useful information in itself.

Note also that during this woman's caloric testing, there are considerable random fluctuations in slow-phase velocity. There seems, in fact, to be a failure of visual suppression during the first (right-cool) caloric. This would have to be considered pathological if consistent. Other segments of the tracings, however, show equally rapid changes in velocity unrelated to eye openings.

Upon rereading this ENG for publication, the variation in caloric nystagmus could also be called dysmetric. While one of the causes for dysmetria is fluctuating alertness, other causes do exist that are related to important pathologies in the posterior fossa and probably elsewhere, including contusions.[12,18]

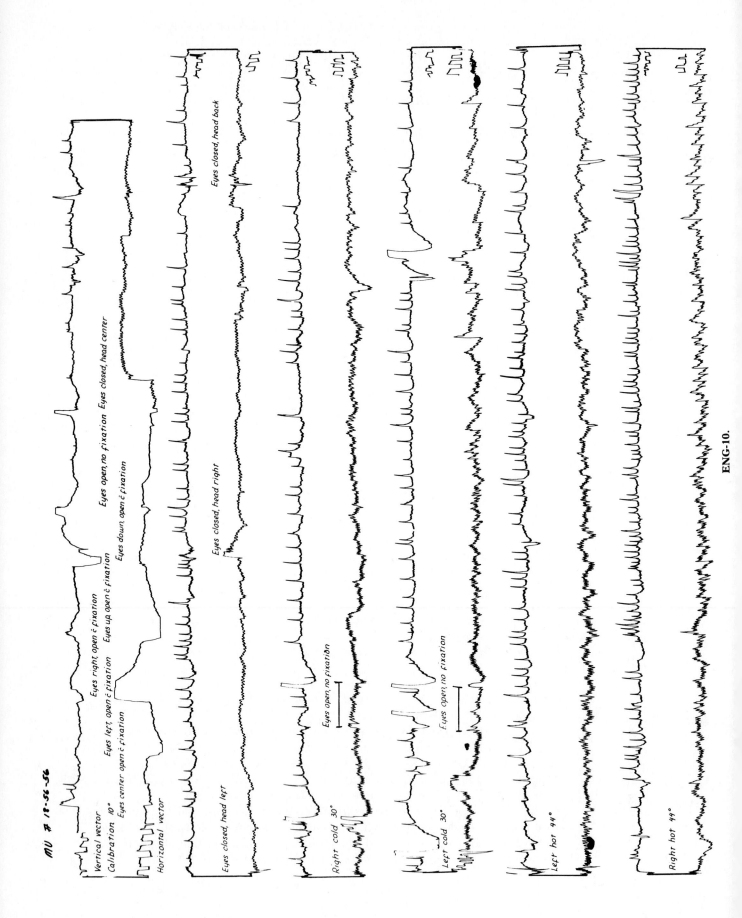

MV # 18-56-56

Vertical vector

Calibration 10°

Eyes center open c̄ fixation

Eyes right, open c̄ fixation   Eyes open, no fixation   Eyes closed, head center

Eyes left, open c̄ fixation

Eyes up open c̄ fixation

Eyes down, open c̄ fixation

Horizontal vector

Eyes closed, head back

Eyes closed, head left

Eyes closed, head right

Right cold 30°

Eyes open, no fixation

Left cold 30°

Eyes open, no fixation

Left hot 44°

Right hot 44°

ENG-10.

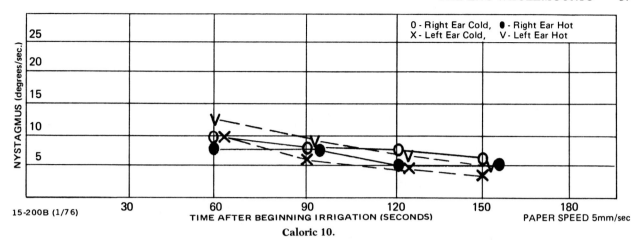

Caloric 10.

15-200B (1/76)

ENG-10

History: This 57-year-old female has a 2- to 3-year history of intermittent "spinning" dizziness, unrelated to body position but increased by rapid positional changes. She complains of tinnitus and a "plugged" sensation in the left ear. Relaxation relieves the dizziness. Her past history includes somatic-tension symptoms and a positive serologic test for syphilis adequately treated with penicillin 1 year ago. Examination and workup are negative except for a very slight low-frequency hearing loss on the left with normal discrimination.

ENG Report: There is no gaze nystagmus. There are very rapid saccadic eye movements when the lids are closed. Its period is approximately 2.4 beats per second, quite regular, and not affected by head motion (see Fig. ENG-10-1).

Bithermal caloric-induced nystagmus is within normal limits for nystagmus velocity and right-left symmetry. The caloric stimulations override this saccadic nystagmus.

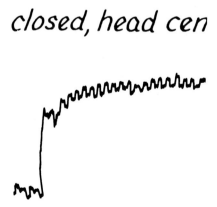

Fig. ENG-10-1. Beginning segment of eyes-closed, head-center tracing.

IMPRESSION.   Normal vestibular examination, plus probably incidental finding of congenital visual system nystagmus.

Comment: The regularly patterned to-and-fro eye movements seen in this tracing are unusual and represent one of several forms of poorly understood visual system defects, usually congenital and typically attributed to the midbrain. This form is not clinically significant. It can be mistaken for a true spontaneous nystagmus, however, if the absence of a fast and a slow component is not detected. One clue that should arouse a reader's suspicions is the very regular period of the eye motion, a feature that is common to most congenital nystagmus.

Most congenital nystagmus is present or most obvious with the eyes open and vision fixed. It is always in the horizontal plane, and there is usually a fixation point slightly off the midline at which the nystagmus may disappear or diminish.[7, 17, 27]

In my experience, these eye motions do not interfere with caloric-induced vestibular nystagmus. In rare cases where there is a vestibular defect causing a nystagmus and also a congenital visual nystagmus, the two eye motions superimpose.

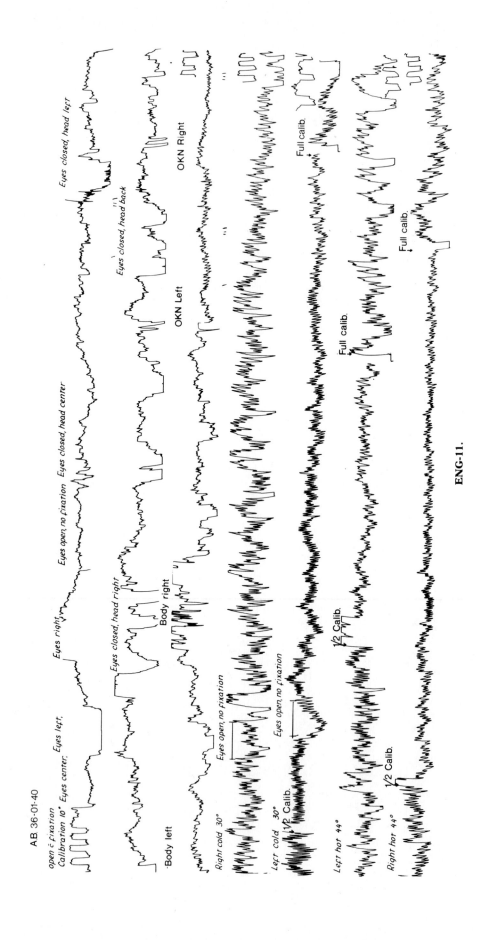

ENG-11.

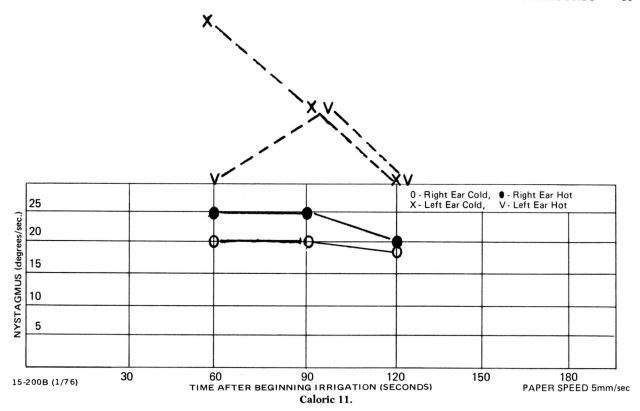

0 - Right Ear Cold, ● - Right Ear Hot
X - Left Ear Cold, V - Left Ear Hot

NYSTAGMUS (degrees/sec.)

25

20

15

10

5

15-200B (1/76)

30   60   90   120   150   180

TIME AFTER BEGINNING IRRIGATION (SECONDS)

PAPER SPEED 5mm/sec

Caloric 11.

ENG-11

History: A 61-year-old female has had intermittent dizzy spells over the past 10 years. Her problem is primarily unsteadiness that occurs every 2 to 5 weeks. Her symptoms are worse in the morning and often associated with nausea, fullness in the ears, subjective hearing loss, and right-sided tinnitus. Until recently her symptoms have been controlled with nicotinic acid. Examination and neurological testing are normal. Audiometry shows a bilateral sensorineural hearing loss, worse on the right. Internal auditory tomograms are normal, as is an ophthalmological examination.

ENG Report: There is a slightly irregular physiological gaze nystagmus. The tracing has an increase in muscle tremor. There is no spontaneous or position-induced nystagmus present, except for a slight right-beating nystagmus with body rotation.

OPN is asymmetrical. Tracking to the left is greater than to the right.

Bithermal caloric-induced nystagmus is asymmetrical. The responses on the right are hypoactive compared to the left.

IMPRESSION. Abnormal examination, asymmetrical OPN, and asymmetrical caloric responses.

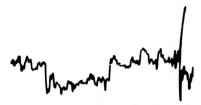

Fig. ENG-11-1.   Segment of eyes-closed, head-center tracing.

Diagnosis: Meniere's syndrome.

Comment: There is considerable muscle tremor in these recordings (see Fig. ENG-11-1) that is not as apparent here as in the original tracings. Most such tremors are normal and indicate only that the patient is highly aroused or "nervous." If continuous throughout the tracing, one need not worry about arousal during caloric tests. In fact, most such patients have accentuated or "hyperactive" responses, as did this woman. I do not usually report calorics as being "hyperactive," since this is only a variation of normal if one can be assured that a very rare midline posterior fossa lesion is not at fault. It is my clinical hunch that "hyperactive" caloric responses usually accompany patients who seem generally overreactive to their symptoms.

The OPN is asymmetrical and probably abnormal (see Fig. ENG-11-2). I have no explanation for this but suspect that the asymmetry was caused by an underlying spontaneous vestibular nystagmus that failed to register in routine testing. Note the intermittent right-beating nystagmus in the lateral head and body

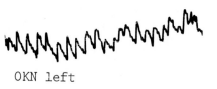

OKN left

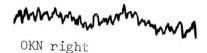

OKN right

Fig. ENG-11-2.   Segments of the left and right OPN responses.

positions. Coats, however, states that a vestibular nystagmus does not create asymmetries in OPN unless the nystagmus has a velocity of at least 5°–7° per second.[9] Unidirectional defects in the absence of a gaze or spontaneous nystagmus can occur from drugs, drowsiness, and rarely with cortical blindness.[26] Ocular defects, most often congenital nystagmus, can also cause such asymmetry, which would have been apparent elsewhere on this test.

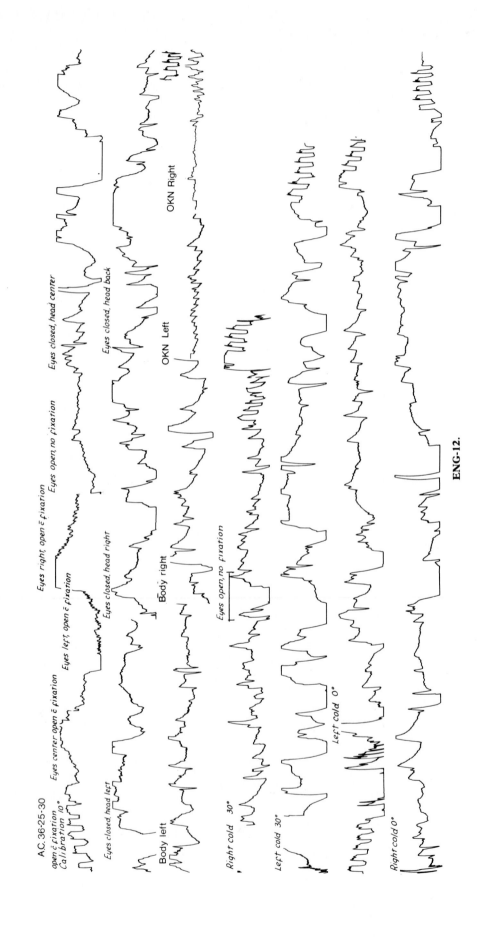

A.C. 36-25-30

Calibration 10°
open c̄ fixation

Eyes center open c̄ fixation

Eyes left, open c̄ fixation

Eyes right, open c̄ fixation

Eyes open, no fixation

Eyes open, no fixation

Eyes closed, head left

Eyes closed, head right

Eyes closed, head center

Eyes closed, head back

Body left

Body right

OKN Left

OKN Right

Right cold 30°

Left cold 30°

Left cold 0°

Right cold 0°

ENG-12.

64

ENG-12

History: A 27-year-old pregnant female has a 6-month history of unsteady gait and blurred vision. She has a 4- to 5-year history of decreased hearing in the right ear, which has acutely worsened in the past 2 weeks. She had an aunt who died of a brain tumor.

Exam shows bilateral papilledema, positive Romberg sign, intention tremor, and upward and lateral gaze nystagmus bilaterally. Cranial nerves V, VII, and IX on the right side are hypoactive. An audiogram shows a profound right sensorineural hearing loss and a mild left loss with positive tone decay. Tomograms show erosion of the right internal auditory canal and a questionable tumor of the left canal.

ENG Report: On calibration tracking, there is a tracking overshoot to the right only. There is a large-amplitude right- and left-gaze nystagmus present. There is a right-beating spontaneous nystagmus present with eyes open without fixation and which is only transiently recordable when the lids are closed. With eyes closed, there is a marked decrement in the fast phase of this transient nystagmus, producing a slow and irregular nystagmus at 3°–5° per second. There are no appreciable positional effects. There are abnormal large shifts of an apparently random nature in recording baseline present during eyes-closed testing. Optokinetic nystagmus is abnormal and asymmetrical.

Cool-water (30° and 0°) stimulation produced no response bilaterally.

IMPRESSION. Abnormal examination, tracking overshoot, gaze nystagmus, spontaneous nystagmus with a possible decrement in its fast phase, abnormal OPN, and no caloric responses.

Diagnosis: Von Recklinghausen's disease was discovered at craniotomy. She had a large acoustic neuroma on the right compressing the cerebellum and a smaller neuroma on the left.

Comment: This ENG confirms the audiometric and neurological findings and is otherwise classical for a posterior fossa defect—calibration overshoots, marked gaze nystagmus, poor OPN responses, and depressed calorics.

Decrements in the speed of the fast or recovery phase of both vestibular and visual nystagmus do occur, although they are not clinically important in this particular case. They are sometimes consistently present and sometimes intermittent. There are several alternative causes, the most common by ENG being an eye motion vector not in the plane of the recording electrodes. Extraocular muscle palsies, drugs, lesions in the pons and brain stem, and occasionally basal ganglia disease are the more common pathological causes.[45]

Note that the baseline wanders widely throughout the recording when the lids are closed. There are three common reasons for this:

1. Random fluctuations in the DC skin potential, usually reflecting changes in the patient's level of arousal (most common cause).
2. Loose electrodes, in which pen swings are often associated with head movement.
3. Bilateral loss of vestibular function with associated loss of vestibular stabilizing of the ocular reflexes with closed lids.

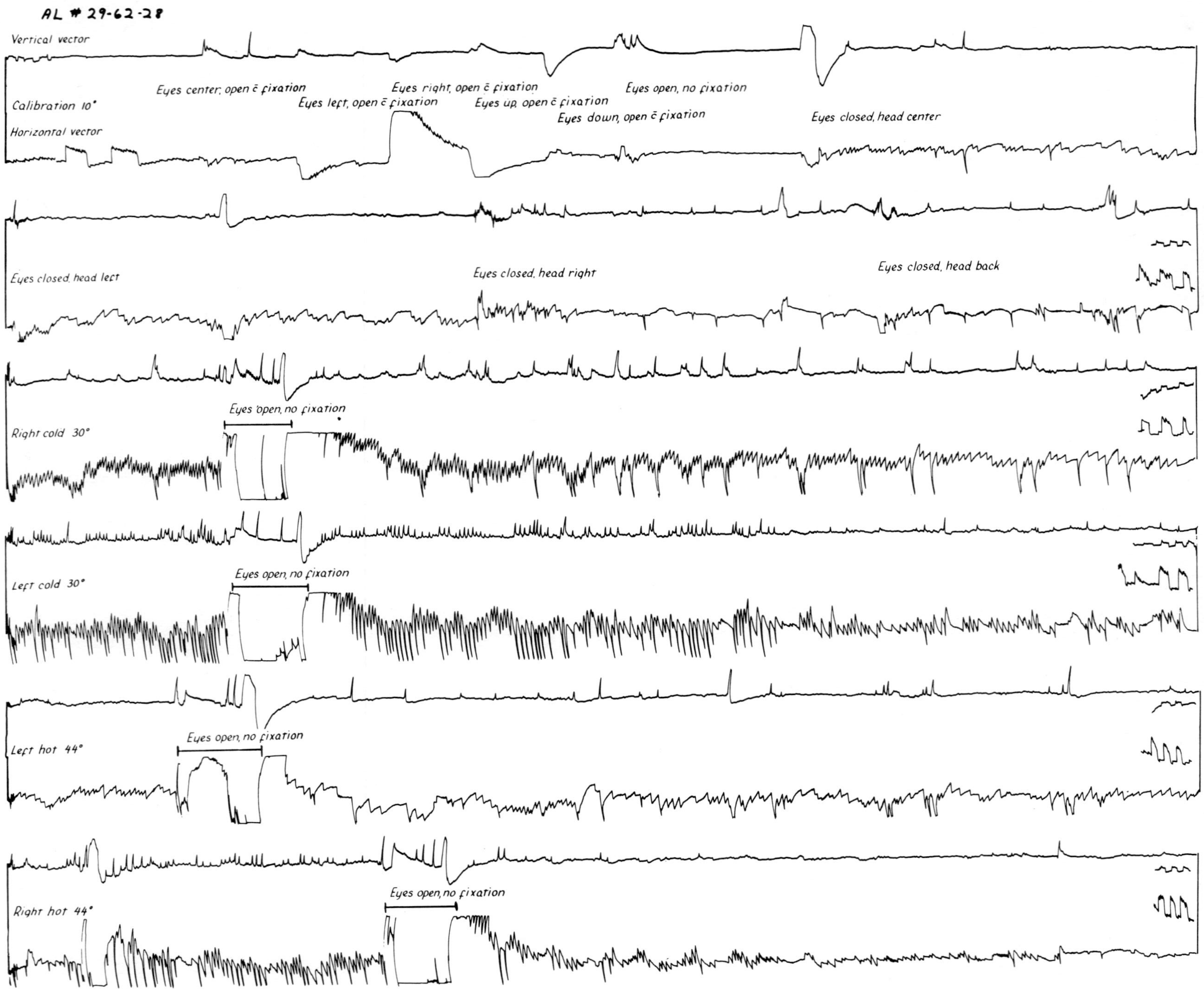

AL # 29-62-28

Vertical vector

Calibration 10°

Horizontal vector

Eyes center, open c̄ fixation

Eyes left, open c̄ fixation

Eyes right, open c̄ fixation

Eyes up, open c̄ fixation

Eyes down, open c̄ fixation

Eyes open, no fixation

Eyes closed, head center

Eyes closed, head left

Eyes closed, head right

Eyes closed, head back

Right cold 30°

Eyes open, no fixation

Left cold 30°

Eyes open, no fixation

Left hot 44°

Eyes open, no fixation

Right hot 44°

Eyes open, no fixation

ENG-13.

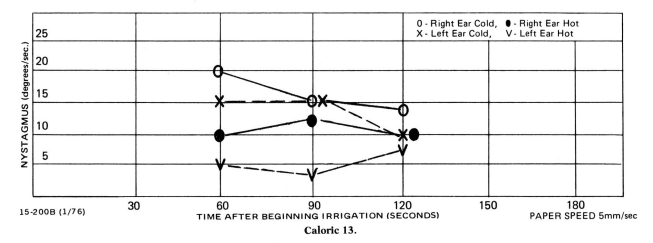

25

20

15

10

5

NYSTAGMUS (degrees/sec.)

0 - Right Ear Cold, ● - Right Ear Hot
X - Left Ear Cold, V - Left Ear Hot

15-200B (1/76)

30   60   90   120   150   180

TIME AFTER BEGINNING IRRIGATION (SECONDS)

PAPER SPEED 5mm/sec

Caloric 13.

ENG-13

History: A 69-year-old female presents with a 5-month history of attacks of dizziness with loss of balance, nausea, and vomiting. She has a history of left-sided high-pitched tinnitus and progressive hearing loss over the past 2 years. Her past history includes a right mastoidectomy 40 years ago and chronic left ear "infections" treated with diphenylhydantoin. She has progressive retinal degeneration (cause not stated) and borderline glaucoma. Examination shows horizontal gaze nystagmus, a normal-appearing left ear, and a negative neurological exam. There is a severe left sensorineural hearing loss, with a discrimination of 4 percent and an SRT of 74 dB. SISI is 100 percent, and tone decay is 20–30 dB in 1 minute.

ENG Report: There is a right and left lateral gaze nystagmus more prominent to the right. There is also a right- and sometimes left-beating fixation nystagmus (Fig. ENG-13-1) and a left-beating spontaneous nystagmus with eyes closed (ap-

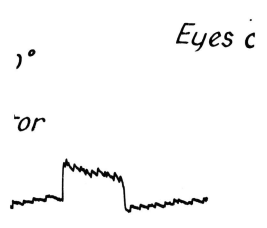

Fig. ENG-13-1. Segment of calibration test.

proximate rate is 5°–8° per second). This nystagmus is decreased in the head-right and head-back positions.

Bithermal caloric-induced nystagmus is asymmetrical. The response to the left-warm caloric is severely hypoactive.

IMPRESSION.   Abnormal examination; fixation, gaze, and spontaneous nystagmus; and hypoactive left-warm caloric.

Diagnosis: Probable Meniere's disease. Follow-up 7 years later shows bilateral progression of hearing loss and no persistent vestibular symptoms. She wears a hearing aid on the right ear. Her retinal degeneration has progressed.

Comment: First note that there is an inadequate electrical signal for 10 mm of pen deflection in the vertical electrodes. This may be related to her retinal degeneration or simply to distance from the eye.

This is an unusual set of eye movements that do not all fit the clinical impression of Meniere's syndrome. Fixation produces a mainly right-beating nystagmus which is accentuated by looking to the right (see calibration tracings, for example). This nystagmus disappears when fixation is prevented.

A bilateral "gaze" nystagmus is also present, and its amplitude toward the right is well outside any physiological range. Normally this would be a strong point in favor of a posterior fossa lesion in a patient with disequilibrium. In this patient, we are probably observing only more fixation nystagmus. Fixation and gaze nystagmus are separate entities, but if a patient with fixation nystagmus also attempts to fixate on the gaze target, nystagmus results. An intranuclear ophthalmoplegia could be causing these same movements, and these differences are not detectable by ENG.

The remainder of the ENG is fairly classical for an end-organ vestibular problem. Note also that there is a consistent tonic deviation of the eyes to the right and down when the lids are closed. Thus, when the eyes are opened and return to the midline during the FFS tests, the pen swings dramatically to the left and then back to the right when the lids are once again closed. Tonic deviation of the closed eyes can be caused by peripheral vestibular abnormalities. Hallpike says deviations of as much as 30° occur, and when there is also a nystagmus preponderance, the deviation is toward the opposite side.[20] In this case the results of the tonic deviation were disastrous for a reading for FFS. Her eyes should have remained open long enough for the time constant of the machine to recenter the pen.

There is also a consistent eye blinking associated with right-beating nystagmus. I do not know its significance. The other nonvestibular visual findings are consistent with retinal degeneration.

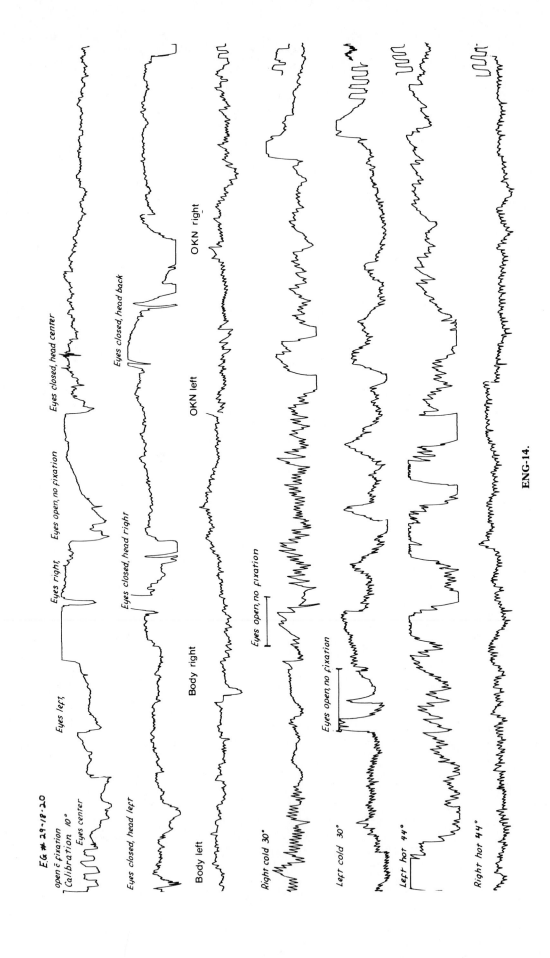

EG # 29-18-20

open c̄ fixation
Calibration 10°
Eyes center

Eyes left,

Eyes right,   Eyes open, no fixation   Eyes closed, head center

Eyes closed head left

Eyes closed, head right   Eyes closed, head back

Body left

Body right   OKN left   OKN right

Right cold 30°   Eyes open, no fixation

Left cold 30°   Eyes open, no fixation

Left hot 44°

Right hot 44°

ENG-14.

70

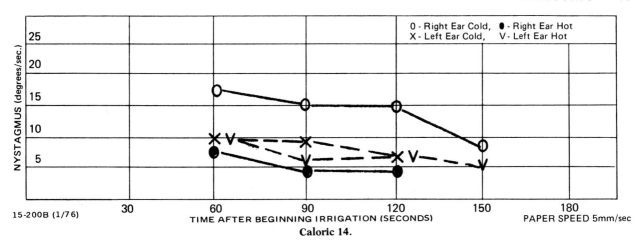

Caloric 14.

15-200B (1/76)

ENG-14

History: A 71-year-old female has had nausea, vomiting, and dizziness for the past week. Three years ago, she had a small myocardial infarction and has had two subsequent hospital admissions for supraventricular tachycardia. For several years, she has complained of staggering and light-headedness, usually related to rapid movement. Repeated neurological examinations and tests for postural hypotension were negative. Fifteen years ago, she had a hemigastrectomy for intractable ulcer pain.

One week ago, she became severely light-headed and nauseated and vomited intractably. Her symptoms are aggravated by standing, and she tends to retropulse on standing. She had orthostatic hypotension. She was treated symptomatically with some improvement. Her symptoms returned within the week, however.

Examination shows an ill-appearing female with essentially normal physical findings. She is not dehydrated and has no neck bruits or fundoscopic changes. Blood pressure is 125/80. Electrolytes are normal. Audiogram shows a bilateral high-frequency hearing loss, recruitment, and no tone decay.

ENG Report: There is no gaze or spontaneous nystagmus. There is a transient right-beating positioning nystagmus on assuming the head-left position and a sustained right-beating nystagmus in the body-right position. OPN tracking is normal.

Caloric-induced nystagmus is asymmetrical and abnormal. Nystagmus to the right has a much different vector than that to the left, and nystagmus to the left is moderately dysrhythmic. There is probably also a nystagmus preponderance to the left, but this is difficult to interpret because of the difficulty in measuring the left-cold and right-warm nystagmus vectors.

IMPRESSION. Abnormal examination, position-induced nystagmus, and asymmetrical caloric-induced nystagmus (see above).

COMMENT. The clinical significance of this caloric vector difference is unclear and could be related to eye muscle imbalance, a peripheral vestibular disorder, or a defect somewhere in between. If clinically indicated, this test should be repeated with direct visual observation.

Diagnosis: Subsequent hospital course yielded a working diagnosis of dizziness secondary to hyponatremia and nausea and vomiting secondary to acute cholecystitis. This was treated symptomatically, and her symptoms were resolved.

Comment: The transient nystagmus occurring immediately after the head-left position is assumed is called a "positioning nystagmus." Normal individuals may show 3 to 5 nystagmus beats upon head positioning. The example here is longer and is probably abnormal.

The caloric abnormalities mentioned in the report are unusual but not rare. The most common cause is an artifact. If the strip-chart pen presses against the paper more firmly in one direction than in the other, an artificial asymmetry results. Usually, one sees this as a rounding of the peaks at the end of the fast phase. A good place to check for this is during the calibrations and OPN tests. If these too are asymmetrical, there is a good chance for an artifact, but remember, a partial or complete ocular muscle paralysis can create these same findings. In this exam, calibrations and OPN are normal. The nystagmus to the right probably has more of a rotary vector than the nystagmus to the left. This should still be checked out visually, however.

Look closely at the head-center, eyes-closed tracing. There seems to be a low-grade nystagmus present. Which way is it beating? Random saccades can occasionally resemble nystagmus, and this is an example. One way to help resolve the question of whether nystagmus is present or absent is to check the directions of the fast phases. Saccades generally have as many to the right as to the left, as in this example.

This woman's subsequent benign clinical course makes all of the above irrelevant here. However, I still suspect that she has either vertebral-basilar artery insufficiency or a partial unilateral labyrinthine defect.

Upper gastrointestinal tract disease, particularly gallbladder trouble, is not an uncommon cause of mild to moderate degrees of dizziness. Such cases do not usually arrive at an ENG laboratory, but they do slip through the medical screens occasionally. Questions about gastrointestinal symptoms in patients with obscure dizziness are worth asking.

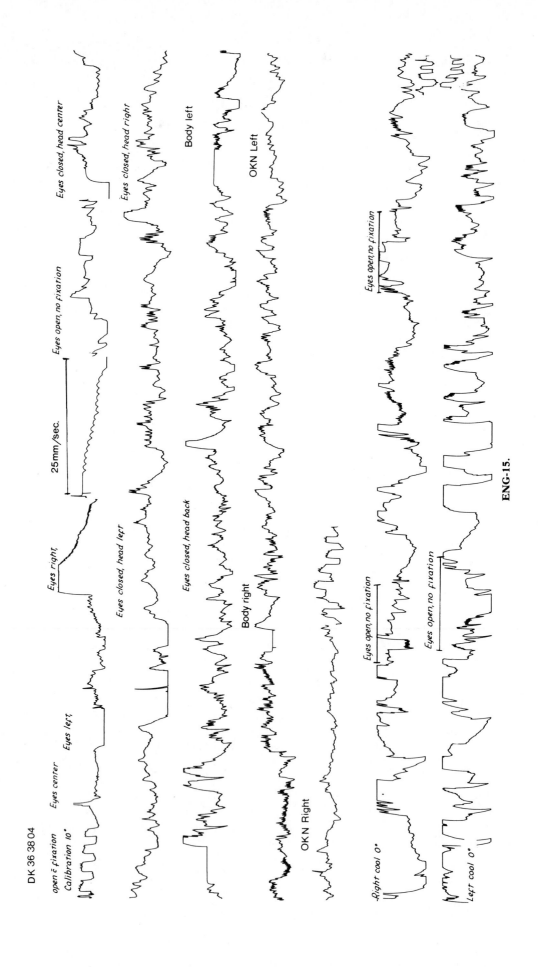

DK 36 38 04

Eyes center   Eyes right,   Eyes closed, head center

open c̄ fixation   Eyes left,   Eyes open, no fixation
Calibration 10°

25mm/sec.

Eyes closed, head left   Eyes closed, head right

Body left

Eyes closed, head back   OKN Left

Body right

OKN Right

Eyes open, no fixation   Eyes open, no fixation

Right cool 0°   Eyes open, no fixation

Left cool 0°

ENG-15.

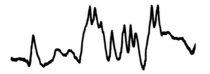

Fig. ENG-15-1. Segment of eyes-closed, head-left tracing.

ENG-15

History: A 47-year-old female has a long-standing history of bilateral hearing loss. She has mild diabetes, well controlled with diet. A younger sister states that the patient has had abnormal eye movements ever since she can remember. Exam shows bilateral gaze nystagmus. Audiogram reveals bilateral combined hearing loss with a 30–40 dB air-bone gap. A diagnosis of otosclerosis was confirmed at tympanotomy.

ENG Report: There is a coarse nystagmus on left lateral gaze and a very rapid fine nystagmus on right gaze. Neither has a definable quick and slow component (see 25 mm/sec paper speed recording). There is possibly an irregular right-beating nystagmus when the eyes are centered without visual fixation, but none present when the lids are closed. There are intermittent bursts of nystagmus, typically without a quick and slow component throughout the positional tests. When these components are identifiable, there is a tendency to beat to the left in the head-left position, to the right in the head-right position, and to the left in the body-left position. I cannot define a vector with body-left, although this position produces the most rapid nystagmus. OPN is bilaterally abnormal. There is no response to ice water calorics in either ear.

IMPRESSION. Abnormal examination, probable congenital visual nystagmus, and no response to caloric stimulations.

Diagnosis: Otosclerosis. Possible congenital fixation nystagmus.

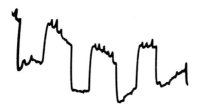

Fig. ENG-15-2. Segment of calibration tracking after OPN testing.

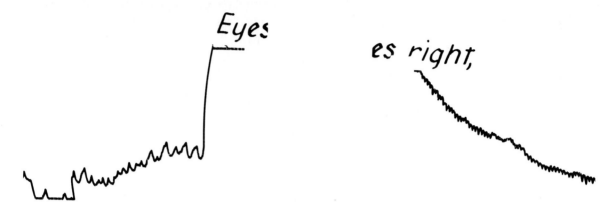

Fig. ENG-15-3 (A and B).   Left- and right-gaze tests.

Comment: This ENG was obtained because the surgeon discovered the gaze nystagmus during his preoperative examination. There was no history of spatial disorientation.

The overall pattern resembles a congenital fixation nystagmus, but not quite. Classical fixation nystagmus disappears completely when the lids are closed. This woman's nystagmus appears and disappears in bursts (see Fig. ENG-15-1) and is also more prominent in some head and body positions than in others. Note also that there is often no quick and slow component.

The "fixation" nystagmus is first observable in the calibration trace to the right (Fig. ENG-15-2) and is not always present. It is more dramatic during gaze testing (Fig. ENG-15-3). This is not a gaze nystagmus. There is no quick and slow component. There is a marked difference in the amplitude and rate of the eyes-left and eyes-right saccades. This, too, is unusual. Typically both directions are symmetrical.

The poor to absent responses to OPN testing are fairly common with congenital visual nystagmus.[9] The absence of caloric responses is very likely real and reflects a true loss of labyrinthine function. Vestibular nystagmus will override a congenital visual nystagmus, although one may have trouble sorting one from the other if the visual nystagmus is also present with eyes closed.

All of the above presupposes that the rather vague history of this patient is correct. Cerebellar degeneration could produce many of these same findings.

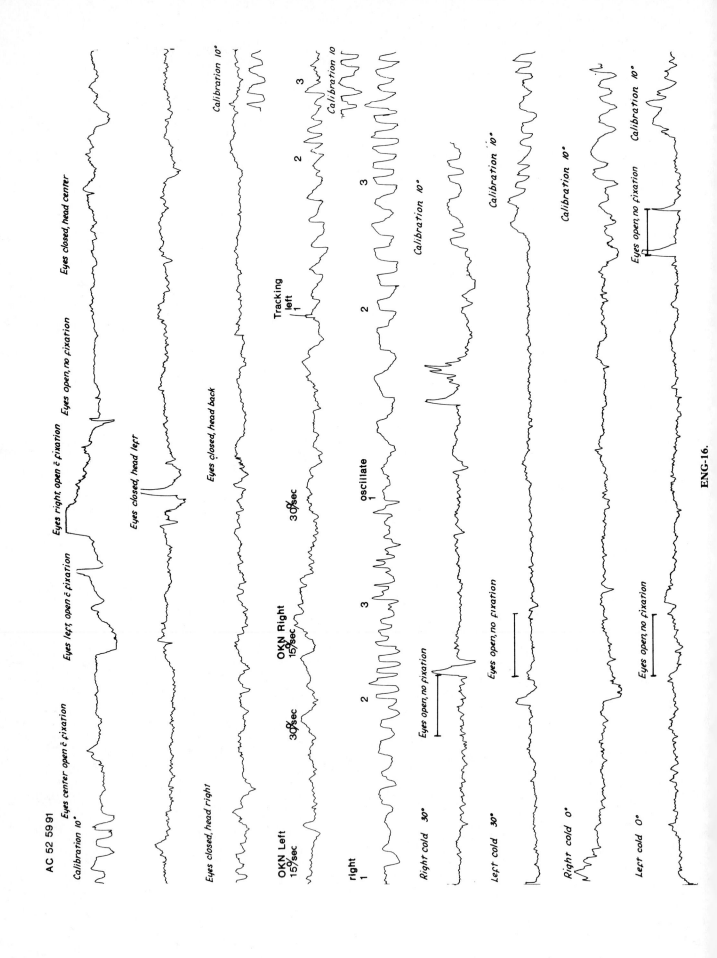

ENG-16.

ENG-16

History: This 65-year-old female has a long history of slowly progressive disequilibrium preceded by loss of color vision. The disequilibrium is not episodic and not associated with nausea, vomiting, or hearing loss. She now requires assistance to walk. She has had slurred speech for the past 5 years and has some problems handling liquid foods. Her brother has a similar problem with disequilibrium and visual deterioration.

Examination shows a wide-based gait and all of her cerebellar tests including finger-to-nose, rapid alternating movements, and Romberg are grossly abnormal. She cannot read 2-cm letters 6 inches away nor can she identify colored cards. There is bilateral ptosis and decreased upward gaze. Otherwise, extraocular muscle function is normal.

ENG Report: Calibration tracking is abnormal, probably secondary to poor vision. A questionably significant right-gaze nystagmus is present. There is no spontaneous or position-induced nystagmus. Optokinetic nystagmus is abnormal (see tracing). Tracking is poor.

Bithermal caloric-induced nystagmus is absent. Additional stimulation with 5 ml of ice water produced a slight response.

IMPRESSION. Abnormal examination, abnormal calibration tracking, abnormal tracking, abnormal OPN, questionable gaze nystagmus, and very hypoactive caloric responses.

Diagnosis: Progressive neurodegenerative disease, possibly Marie's ataxia.

Comment: Most ENGs are interpretable without knowing the clinical history and findings of the patient. This one is not. On cursory examination of the eye movement tracings, none of the stimuli—visual tracking, body positioning, OPNs, or calorics—seem to elicit expected responses. Nothing seems to be working quite right. This woman has both attenuated visual and vestibular function. She cannot see to track the calibration lights.* Furthermore, it was necessary to increase the recorder gain to near maximum to obtain 10 mm of pen deflection for the approximate 10° of eye movement. The corneoretinal potential was markedly attenuated. This sometimes occurs normally in some elderly individuals and more commonly in persons with retinal degeneration at any age.

The visual defect might be entirely peripheral, but the OPNs are also grossly abnormal, and even a nearly blind person ought to perform normally with the very easy OPN stimulus. Thus, a peripheral visual problem is not the only defect. The bilateral OPN defect is almost certainly cerebellar in origin.[44] There is also severe depression of all caloric responses. This hypoactivity is probably real, but when the visual system is also abnormal, there is no way to determine if the calorics' failure to produce nystagmus results from defective end-organs or from a defective visual system reflection of the vestibular input.

As exemplified here, pursuit-tracking tasks in patients with poor peripheral vision are futile. If the stimuli are not seen, they cannot be tracked.

---

* Reasonably good calibration in blind persons can be obtained by using proprioceptive cues. Ask the patient to visually follow his thumb as it is moved 10° to the right and then 10° to the left.

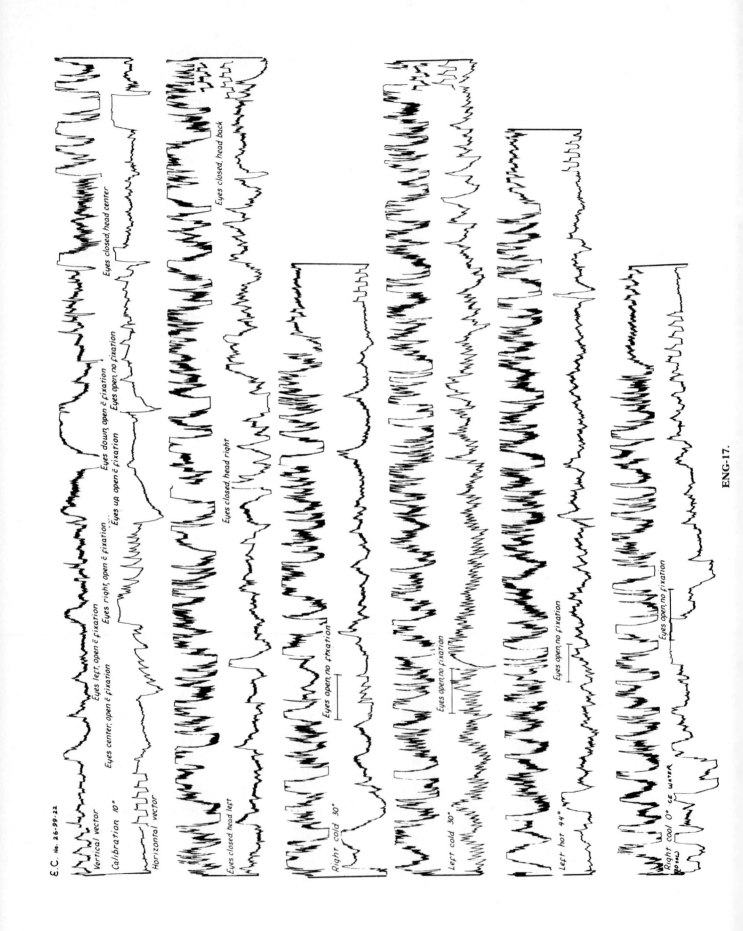

E.C. No. 26-99-22

Vertical vector

Calibration 10°

Horizontal vector

Eyes left, open c̄ fixation

Eyes center, open c̄ fixation

Eyes down, open c̄ fixation

Eyes right, open c̄ fixation

Eyes up, open c̄ fixation

Eyes open, no fixation

Eyes closed, head center

Eyes closed, head left

Eyes closed, head right

Eyes closed, head back

Eyes open, no fixation

Right cold 30°

Eyes open, no fixation

Left cold 30°

Eyes open, no fixation

Left hot 44°

Eyes open, no fixation

Right cool 0° ice water

Eyes open, no fixation

ENG-17.

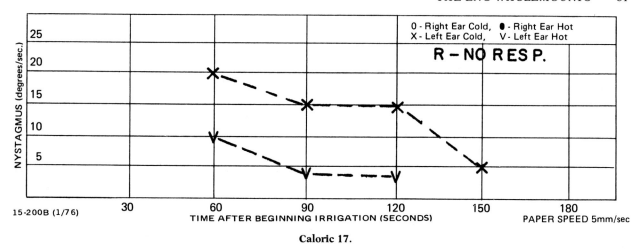

Caloric 17.

ENG-17

History: A 26-year-old male has a 2-month history of right infraorbital numbness, difficulty in walking and speaking, occipital headaches, and vomiting without nausea. He has also developed diplopia and a tremor of the right hand. He complains of a right-sided progressive hearing loss over 2 years. He denies tinnitus and vertigo. Physical examination shows bilateral papilledema with extensive hemorrhages. A brain scan shows increased uptake beneath the cerebellum on the right, and the right internal auditory canal is markedly enlarged on tomograms. There is a severe sensorineural hearing loss on the right, 0 percent discrimination, positive tone decay, no recruitment, and type III Békésy tracking.

ENG Report: There is a significant overshoot defect in visual tracking on the ENG calibrations. There is a large bilateral gaze nystagmus.
  There is a considerable amount of muscle noise and irregular saccades in the recording but no distinct spontaneous or position-induced nystagmus.
  Bithermal caloric-induced nystagmus is abnormal. There is no response on the right side, even with 5 ml of ice water stimulation.

  IMPRESSION. Abnormal examination, marked lateral gaze nystagmus, no response to caloric stimulation of the right ear, and a visual tracking defect (probably cerebellar) to the right.

Diagnosis: A large right acoustic neuroma was found at surgery. Postoperatively, he has a right seventh nerve deficit, a decreased right corneal reflex, and decreased strength of the right arm.

Comment: There are two very firm signs of a posterior fossa defect in this ENG—the calibration overshoot and the very coarse gaze nystagmus. The detail of the calibration overshoot is shown in Fig. ENG-17-1 and represents a dysmetria of the extraocular muscles that can be unidirectional or bidirectional (left, right, or both left and right). As a physical finding, it is most closely correlated with the standard finger-to-nose test. In this instance, the eye "overshoots" the calibration

)n   10°

vector

Fig. ENG-17-1.   Segment of initial calibration.

target in the same manner that the finger overshoots the nose. Such an overshoot can occur in a normal examination but is not consistently present. In order to score it as a positive sign, it must be consistent and present in at least two places on the ENG, excluding the calibrations following the calorics. (Following caloric stimulation, such an overshoot is not at all unusual in normals.) Overshoots must also be distinguished from eye blinks or faulty time constants on the ENG machine itself.[21]

The very coarse gaze nystagmus is also typical for cerebellar lesions. This particular gaze nystagmus happens to be virtually diagnostic if drug effects can be excluded.

There is considerable muscle artifact in this recording, especially in the vertical electrodes. While one frequently sees much more such artifacts in vertical electrodes, the amount here makes these leads almost useless. Be suspicious of the common reference (forehead) electrode when this much muscle artifact appears in both sets of electrodes.

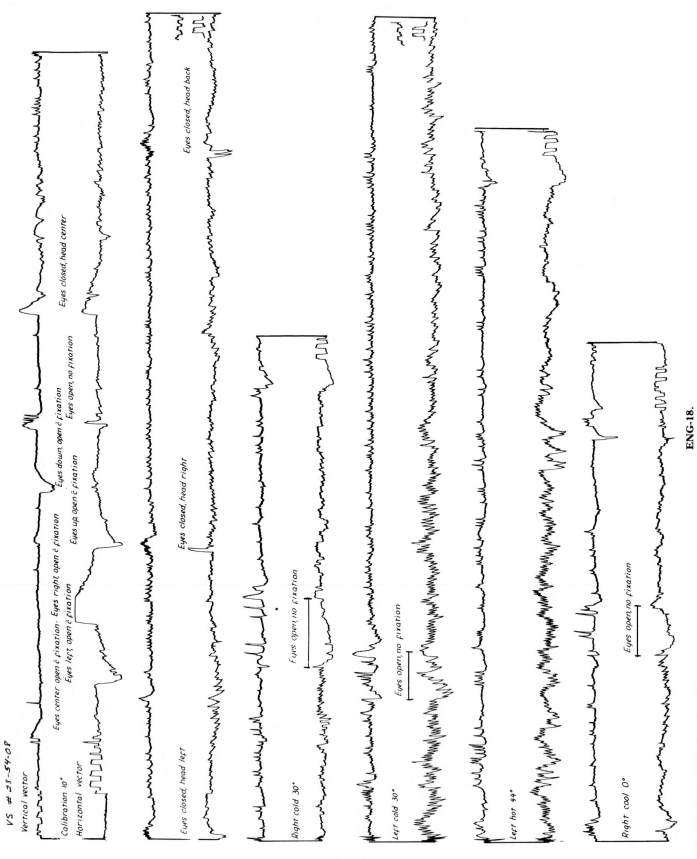

VS # 28-54-08

Vertical vector

Calibration 10°

Horizontal vector

Eyes center open c̄ fixation · Eyes right open c̄ fixation

Eyes left, open c̄ fixation

Eyes down, open c̄ fixation

Eyes up, open c̄ fixation

Eyes closed, head center

Eyes open, no fixation

Eyes open, no fixation

Eyes closed, head back

Eyes closed, head left

Eyes closed, head right

Right cold 30°

Eyes open, no fixation

Left cold 30°

Eyes open, no fixation

Left hot 44°

Right cool 0°

Eyes open, no fixation

ENG-18.

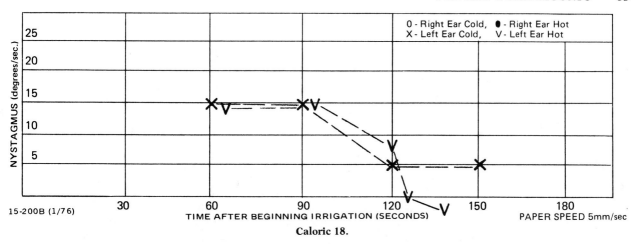

Caloric 18.

ENG-18

History: A 52-year-old female presents with a progressive right-sided hearing loss over the last 4 to 5 years. She denies tinnitus, vertigo, and loss of balance. She has had recent recurrent temporal headaches. Examination shows a decreased right corneal reflex, right facial weakness, a lateral gaze nystagmus, and an ataxic tandem gait. There is no hearing in the right ear. Further workup reveals a mass lesion in the right posterior fossa with obstructive hydrocephalus.

ENG Report: There is a left-gaze nystagmus. There is a slight left-beating spontaneous nystagmus with eyes open, no fixation, which increases with the eyes closed (rate, 3°–5° per second). This changes to a more rapid right-beating nystagmus with head-left position and returns to a left-beating nystagmus with head-right position. During the head-right testing, the nystagmus abruptly and "spontaneously" changes to right-beating, and this same effect can be seen during the right-cold caloric and ice water caloric.

Bithermal caloric-induced nystagmus is abnormal. There is no response to caloric stimulation of the right ear, including 5 ml of ice water.

IMPRESSION. Abnormal examination, gaze nystagmus, direction-changing spontaneous nystagmus which is also affected by head position, and no response to right ear calorics.

Diagnosis: This patient had a "transitional meningioma" arising from the clivus and extending to the right cerebellopontine angle.

Comment: There is one very important finding on this ENG—the direction-changing, position-influenced spontaneous nystagmus. Any nystagmus that changes direction spontaneously indicates a significant central nervous system defect, almost always in the brain stem or cerebellar pathways. When present, even if there are no other signs or findings, it is sufficient to initiate a full-scale neurological evaluation[33] (see ENG-19).

Note that this directional change also occurs during the right calorics. It might be tempting to describe this as a so-called "perverted" caloric nystagmus (one that beats the wrong way). I have never seen a perverted nystagmus that could not be explained by underlying circumstances, such as in this example, and more commonly, by an arousal effect on a latent spontaneous nystagmus.

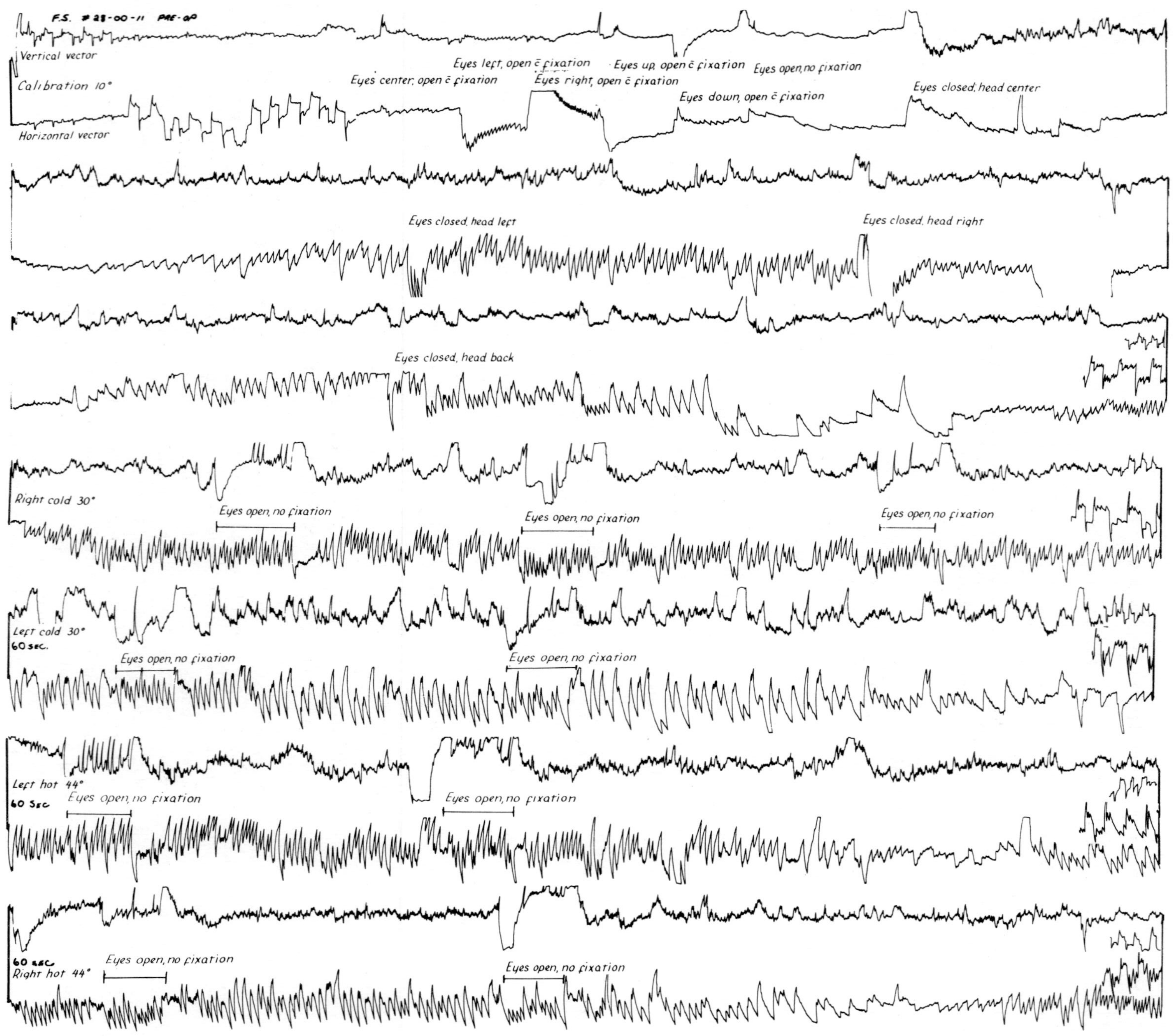

F.S. #21-00-11 PRE-OP

Vertical vector

Calibration 10°

Horizontal vector

Eyes left, open c̄ fixation   Eyes up, open c̄ fixation   Eyes open, no fixation

Eyes center, open c̄ fixation   Eyes right, open c̄ fixation

Eyes down, open c̄ fixation

Eyes closed, head center

Eyes closed, head right

Eyes closed, head left

Eyes closed, head back

Eyes open, no fixation

Right cold 30°

Eyes open, no fixation

Left cold 30°
60 sec.

Eyes open, no fixation

Eyes open, no fixation

Eyes open, no fixation

Left hot 44°
60 sec

Eyes open, no fixation

60 sec
Right hot 44°

Eyes open, no fixation

ENG-19.

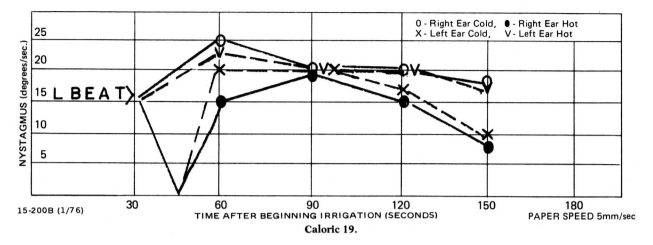

Caloric 19.

ENG-19

History: A 28-year-old male complained of an 8-year history of intermittent spatial disorientation and a "whirling" sensation with rapid changes in head position, initially diagnosed as Meniere's disease. Three years ago, he had an episode of postural vertigo in Africa followed by "meningoencephalitis." Five months ago the patient first noticed intermittent suboccipital headaches and increased postural vertigo and diplopia. When he presented to the neurologist he complained of unsteadiness of gait, occasional diplopia, and two episodes of nasal regurgitation. Examination showed gaze nystagmus, saccadic eye movements on tracking, a question of vertical nystagmus on downward gaze, a right trigeminal hypesthesia, and a slight right facial weakness. Hearing was normal.

ENG Report: This patient has a visual tracking overshoot on the 10° calibration markers and a marked and relatively coarse gaze nystagmus in all except the vertical upward direction. There is a spontaneous nystagmus that beats weakly to the left during visual fixation, then to the right with the eyes open without fixation, and then strongly to the left with the lids closed. This latter, eyes-closed spontaneous nystagmus has a delayed onset of 10 to 20 seconds. It is affected by head position. There is probably a spontaneous directional change during head positioning, but not of the type typically called a position-induced, direction-changing nystagmus. In head-right position, it continues to the left for 20 seconds and then reverses and beats to the right at about the same rate. In the head-back position, it beats to the right for 40 to 50 seconds and then reverses back to the left.

Both ears do respond to caloric stimulation, but because of the vagaries of his superimposed spontaneous nystagmus, symmetry of responses is impossible to determine. There was, for example, an unexplained shift to a spontaneous right-beating nystagmus following the left-warm stimulation. This was accentuated during the right-warm stimulation but reverted to a left-beating nystagmus afterwards.

IMPRESSION.   Abnormal examination, for several reasons. This is almost a classic set of findings for a cerebellar defect or a very unusual congenital lesion, location undetermined.

Diagnosis: The patient had a large midline arachnoidal cyst of the cisterna magna. He did well postoperatively. The "meningoencephalitis" is believed by the neurosurgeons to have represented a previous rupture of the cyst with meningeal inflammation.

Comment: This ENG displays several characteristics of a posterior fossa deficit. The first of these is the consistent overshoot on the calibration tracking. Second is the obvious coarse gaze nystagmus in both lateral directions and vertically in the eyes-down position. Third, there is a highly unusual spontaneous nystagmus present. It is affected by head position, but more importantly, it changes directions spontaneously. This behavior is a fairly classic form of a Nylen type III nystagmus.[34] This one is always characteristic of a central nervous system deficit.

Note also that during the warm caloric testing, the initial nystagmus response is perfectly appropriate, and then as this response decays, the spontaneous nystagmus reappears, beating in the direction opposite to the caloric effect. This phenomenon can be seen in normals but not to this degree. It has been called a "phase II," "secondary," or "after" nystagmus.

There is some confusion in the literature on the significance of type III nystagmus, mainly because all positional nystagmus that does not fit the definitions for type I (direction-changing, position-induced) or type II (direction-fixed, position-influenced) are lumped in the type III group.

Note that there is at least a 30-second onset delay in the spontaneous nystagmus after the lids are closed (eyes-closed, head-center). Such delayed onsets are said to be caused by CNS abnormalities. This is debatable. However, the fact that these delays do occur is good reason to insist on at least a 40-second period of recording.

Failure of fixation suppression during the caloric tests is probably also present.

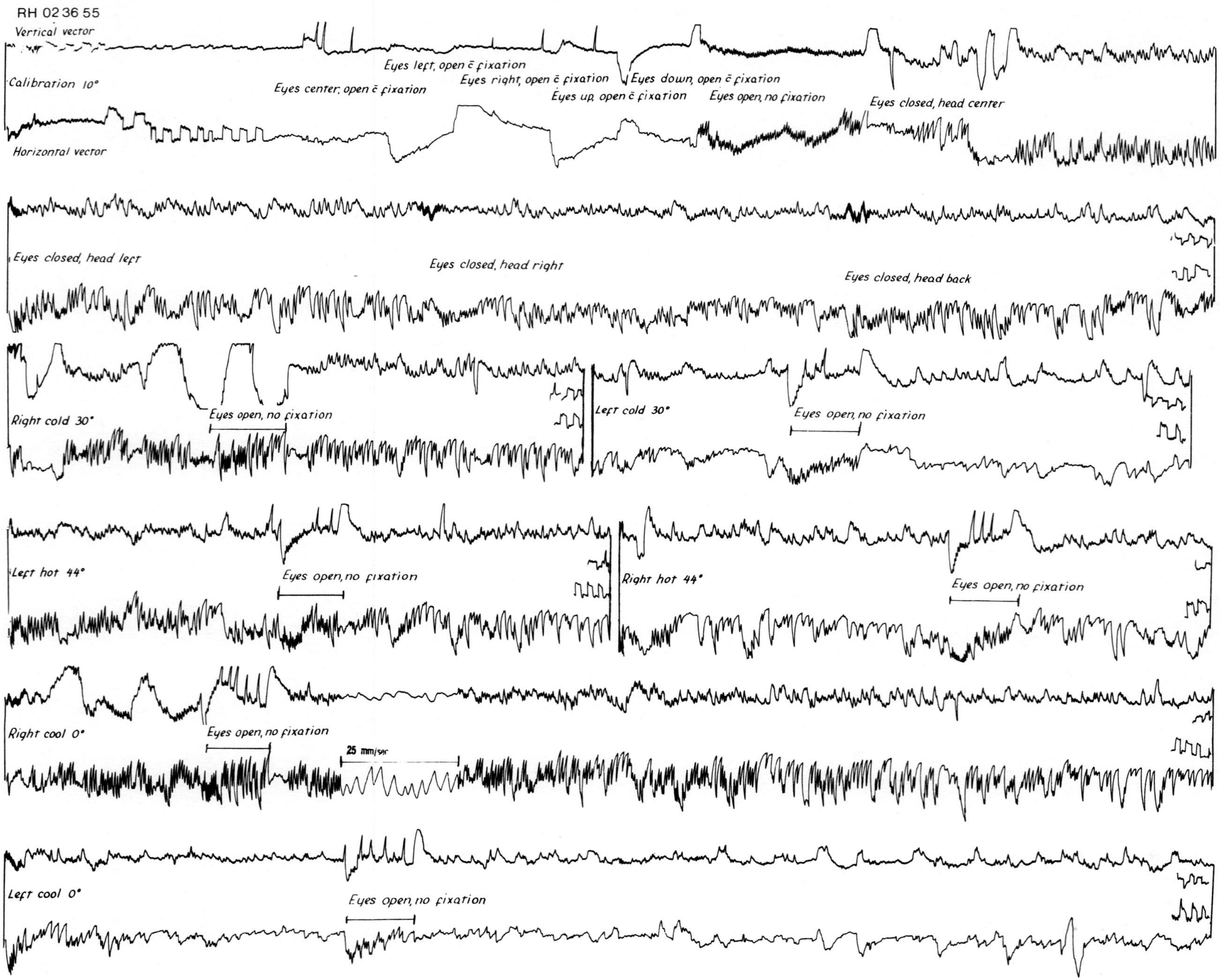

RH 02 36 55

Vertical vector

Calibration 10°

Horizontal vector

Eyes left, open c̄ fixation

Eyes center, open c̄ fixation

Eyes right, open c̄ fixation

Eyes down, open c̄ fixation

Eyes up, open c̄ fixation

Eyes open, no fixation

Eyes closed, head center

Eyes closed, head back

Eyes closed, head right

Eyes closed, head left

Right cold 30°

Left cold 30°

Eyes open, no fixation

Eyes open, no fixation

Left hot 44°

Right hot 44°

Eyes open, no fixation

Eyes open, no fixation

Right cool 0°

25 mm/sec

Eyes open, no fixation

Eyes open, no fixation

Left cool 0°

Eyes open, no fixation

ENG-20.

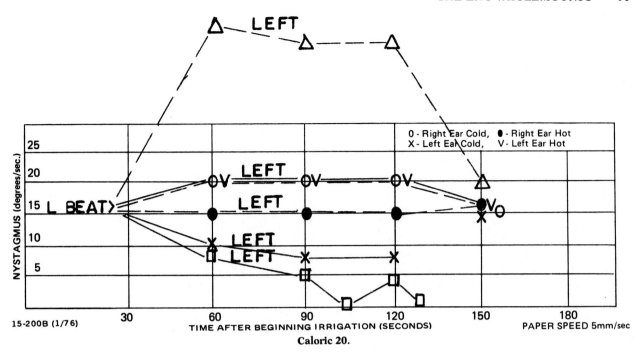

Caloric 20.

15-200B (1/76)

ENG-20

History: A 26-year-old male is referred for evaluation of an 8-month history of intermittent dizziness characterized by light-headedness, mild ataxia, nausea, and vomiting. The onset of an attack is abrupt, the cessation is gradual, and the attacks last from 1 to 6 hours. During the attack, if the patient looks at an object, it may jump back and forth as if he had nystagmus. He also notes a slight "through a funnel"-type of hearing sensation. On two occasions he has noted a disturbance of the function of his right hand. After the attack, he feels completely normal except for mild fatigue. From childhood, he has had a stable left-sided visual and auditory defect attributed to maternal rubella. Examination today shows no ataxia or nystagmus. There is a profound left sensorineural hearing loss with no discrimination and no tone decay.

ENG Report: There is a bilateral gaze nystagmus, probably physiological. There is a marked spontaneous left-beating nystagmus, which is almost inhibited by visual fixation (Fig. ENG-20-1) but is unusually prominent with the eyes open without fixation (Fig. ENG-20-2). With the eyes closed, the amplitude increases, but the slow-phase velocity remains about the same (10°–20° per second) (Fig. ENG-20-3). This nystagmus is modestly decreased with the head to the right.

Bithermal caloric-induced nystagmus shows both labyrinths to be functioning, but the exact calculations of the slow-phase velocity are extremely difficult because of the high-level background of spontaneous nystagmus. The response to right ice

Eyes ce

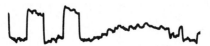

Fig. ENG-20-1. Segments of the initial horizontal calibration and eyes center with visual fixation tests.

water stimulation is probably greater than that to the left. There is an apparent failure of suppression of the caloric nystagmus by opening the eyes (but see Comment).

IMPRESSION.   Abnormal examination, spontaneous left-beating vestibular nystagmus slightly affected by head position, and bilaterally functioning labyrinths (see above).

Comment: This is a highly unusual set of eye movements which follows almost none of the usual patterns for either a peripheral or central defect. This man had an impressive spontaneous nystagmus, yet he was not dizzy during the ENG. This alone would normally rule out a peripheral labyrinthine defect. Visual fixation does inhibit this nystagmus, but "eyes open, no fixation" does not. The only change with "eyes closed" is a larger amplitude, not the expected sizable increment in slow-phase velocity. The "physiological gaze nystagmus" is probably irrelevant, but I would normally expect to see a unilateral gaze nystagmus in the direction of the fast phase of the spontaneous nystagmus, especially if a peripheral lesion is at fault (see ENG-3, for example).

The patient's experience of seeing objects jump back and forth during his attacks is quite uncommon. Normally, cortical vision is inhibited by the superior colliculus during saccades (fast phase of nystagmus). Thus the room or objects do not jump in the visual field but appear to be moving steadily.

Eyes open,

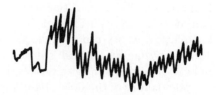

Fig. ENG-20-2.   Eyes open, no fixation.

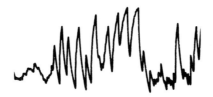

Fig. ENG-20-3.   Eyes-closed, head-center position.

Interpreting the caloric responses is partly guesswork and is based solely on effects that the stimuli might have had on the left-beating spontaneous nystagmus. In the most extreme case (ice water), there is a distinct effect from the right ear—an increase in the left nystagmus with a return to baseline at about 150 seconds. Stimulation of the left ear seems to suppress the spontaneous nystagmus, but the response does not return to baseline as it should. Responses to the other four tests are within the range of variation of the spontaneous nystagmus and are unreliable. This patient should have been retested, with visual fixation maintained during calorics.

The increase in nystagmus during all the calorics when the eyes are open without fixation could be mistaken for a failure of fixation suppression (FFS). This interpretation is incorrect.

Note that during right-beating calorics (left-cold and right-hot) the burst of nystagmus with *eyes open, no fixation* is to the *left*. The best example is during left 0° irrigation. True FFS is an accentuation of the caloric-induced nystagmus by light and visual fixation, and this tracing shows the release of a spontaneous nystagmus.

The most parsimonious explanation of this ENG is two pathologies, one long-standing (perhaps from childhood) within the CNS and a second related to his more recent symptoms. The spontaneous nystagmus is most likely central vestibular and only grudgingly responsive to peripheral stimuli. I have also seen ENGs as wild as this one in patients with Meniere's syndrome, shortly after an attack. Repeating this examination in 1 month would be highly desirable. Interpreting this ENG without a personal examination of this patient is impossible.

Follow-up: Subsequent neurological consultations found nothing else. He was alive and well 1 year later but still having dizzy attacks.

PROBABLE DIAGNOSIS.   Meniere's syndrome with old left-sided congenital CNS defect.

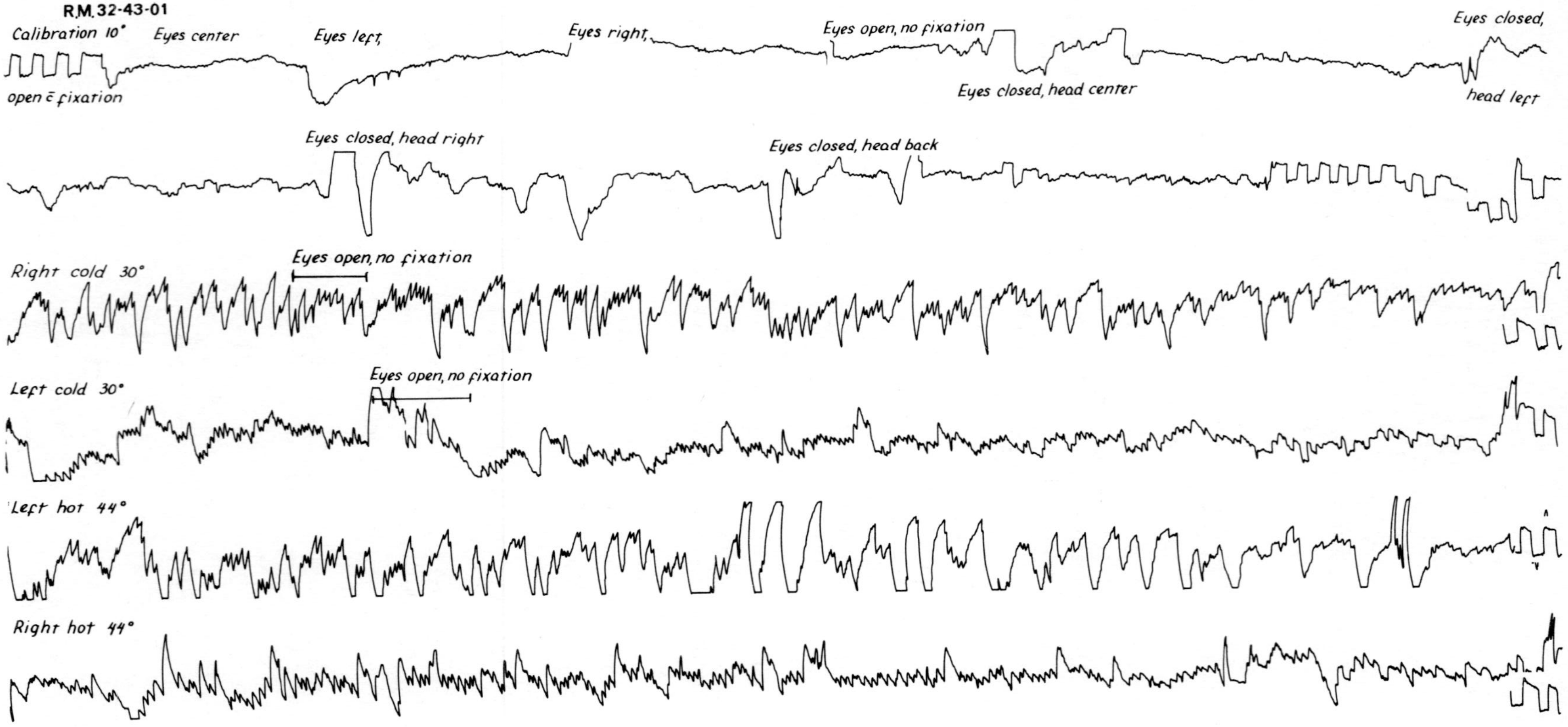

RM.32-43-01

Calibration 10° Eyes center Eyes left, Eyes right, Eyes open, no fixation Eyes closed,

open ē fixation

head left

Eyes closed, head center

Eyes closed, head right

Eyes closed, head back

Right cold 30°

Eyes open, no fixation

Left cold 30°

Eyes open, no fixation

Left hot 44°

Right hot 44°

ENG-21.

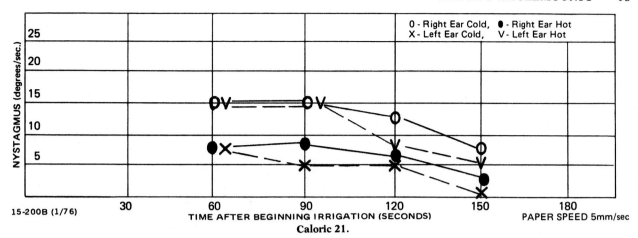

15-200B (1/76)

TIME AFTER BEGINNING IRRIGATION (SECONDS)

PAPER SPEED 5mm/sec

Caloric 21.

ENG-21

History: A 49-year-old male complained of recurrent vertigo. One and one-half years earlier, he had the abrupt onset of vertigo without nausea or vomiting which lasted for several minutes and subsided spontaneously. He was well for a year and then similar episodes started almost weekly. The attacks were not precipitated by movement or change in position, and there was no change in hearing or tinnitus. The patient felt he had difficulty concentrating and was somewhat more forgetful than usual; otherwise there were no focal neurologic signs. A trial on diphenylhydantoin had no effect, and later on he developed slightly slurred speech which disappeared subsequently.

Examination was normal, including cranial and peripheral nerves and auscultation of head and neck. An EEG showed minimal slowing over both temporal lobes. Arteriography showed a hypoplastic left internal carotid and stenosis of the left vertebral artery with reflux filling of the right vertebral artery.

ENG Report: There is no gaze, spontaneous, or position-induced nystagmus present with eyes open or closed.

Bithermal caloric-induced nystagmus is asymmetrical. There is a directional preponderance for the left-going stimuli. There is a significant dysrhythmia of the nystagmus beating to the left.

IMPRESSION.   Abnormal examination and caloric nystagmus preponderance to the left associated with dysrhythmia.

Diagnosis: Vertebral-basilar artery insufficiency.

Follow-up: Six years later the patient is alive and well. He is asymptomatic without treatment.

Comment: Nystagmus preponderance and symmetrical dysrhythmia are both nonspecific ENG abnormalities. When a dysrhythmia is not arousal-related, however, as in this example, it is an important abnormality worth pursuing.[12, 37] This patient most probably had a tonic deviation of his eyes behind closed lids, with a resultant "interference" with the fast phase of nystagmus. There are not enough transitions between eyes open and eyes closed on the tracing to verify the direction of this tonic deviation. OPN responses would probably have been symmetrical if they had been tested.

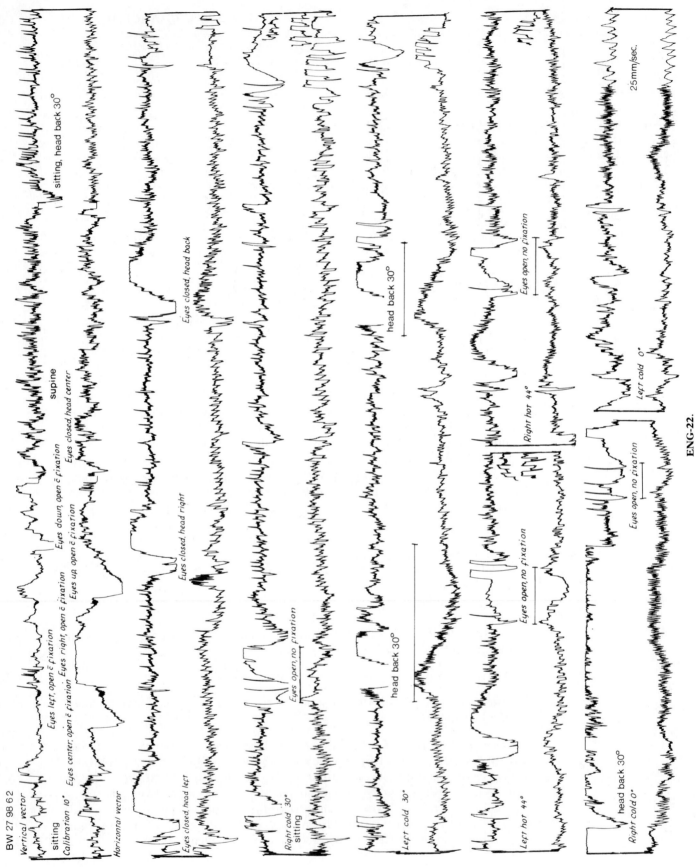

BW 27 98 62

Vertical vector

sitting

Calibration 10°

Eyes center, open c̄ fixation

Eyes left, open c̄ fixation

Eyes right, open c̄ fixation

Eyes down, open c̄ fixation

Eyes up open c̄ fixation

Eyes closed, head center

supine

Horizontal vector

Eyes closed head left

Eyes closed, head back

Eyes closed head right

Right cold 30°

sitting

Eyes open, no fixation

Left cold 30°

head back 30°

head back 30°

Left hot 44°

Right hot 44°

Eyes open, no fixation

Eyes open, no fixation

head back 30°

Right cold 0°

Eyes open, no fixation

Left cold 0°

25mm/sec.

ENG-22.

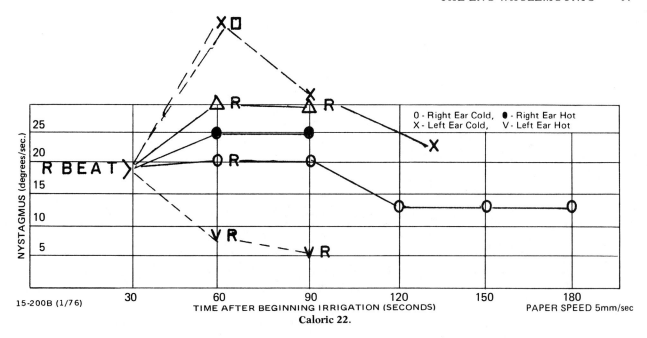

15-200B (1/76)

NYSTAGMUS (degrees/sec.)

R BEAT

0 - Right Ear Cold,   ● - Right Ear Hot
X - Left Ear Cold,   V - Left Ear Hot

TIME AFTER BEGINNING IRRIGATION (SECONDS)
Caloric 22.

PAPER SPEED 5mm/sec

ENG-22

History: This 15-year-old female was admitted to the hospital because of 3 weeks of nausea and vertigo. Two years previously, she had had weakness in her right leg, right arm, and face, along with sensory disturbances in the same areas. EEG, brain scan, and lumbar puncture were all normal at that time. She recovered spontaneously. Since that time, she has had four similar episodes, all resolving within a few days. Three weeks ago, she suddenly developed persistent nausea, imbalance, persistent vertigo (best relieved by lying on her right side), blurred vision, and oscillopsia.

Examination showed conjugate nystagmus in all directions of gaze and a fine nystagmus to the right in central gaze. She had a wide-based gait, truncal and limb ataxia, and incoordination. An ophthalmology consultant noted bilateral retrobulbar neuritis. An audiogram was normal. CSF showed normal protein concentration with increased alpha and beta fractions.

ENG Report: (*Note:* This patient could not be tested in the routine manner because assuming the supine position, especially head-center and head-left, caused her to become vertiginous and nauseated. These symptoms were present in her clinical history and had been continuous for about 2 weeks. If the head-left position was assumed and stabilized, however, the nausea passed in 2 to 3 minutes. The majority of the tests today were obtained with the patient in the sitting position.)

There is a considerable amount of muscle tremor and eye blinking throughout this tracing, which limits the precision of describing other eye movements. There is ocular dysmetria during calibration tracking (Fig. ENG-22-1) and probably a fine left nystagmus during visual fixation (Fig. ENG-22-2). There is an upward gaze nystagmus, but none observable in the other three gaze positions.

There is a right-upward-beating spontaneous nystagmus present with the lids closed (average lateral velocity, 10°–13° per second), which becomes modified to

Calibration 10°

Horizontal vector

Fig. ENG-22-1.   Segment of initial horizontal calibrations.

an almost pure horizontal nystagmus with the head tilted back 30°. It is moderately suppressed in the head-right position.

Evaluation of caloric-induced nystagmus is difficult because of eye-blink artifact and the underlying spontaneous nystagmus. There is probably a response to the left stimulations but very little, if any, response on the right side, even with ice water.

IMPRESSION.   Abnormal examination, ocular dysmetria, upward gaze nystagmus, spontaneous nystagmus affected by head position, and severely hypoactive right caloric responses.

NOTE.   This is a technically difficult tracing to read, and I would suggest a repeat examination if clinically indicated in about 1 month for better detail.

Diagnosis: Multiple sclerosis.

Follow-up: The patient continued to have exacerbations of her disease but was controlled somewhat on ACTH. A repeat ENG was obtained 2 years later using hyperthermia. An increase in body temperature in some patients with multiple sclerosis will produce or increase neurological findings that are missing or borderline at normal body temperature. This is also true for ENG abnormalities.[41] This second ENG was essentially normal except for accentuated saccades.

Eyes center, op

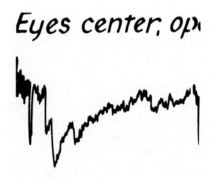

Fig. ENG-22-2.   Eyes center, open with fixation.

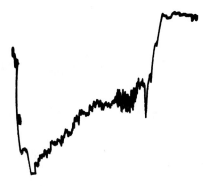

Fig. ENG-22-3. Left-gaze test.

Comment: While the diagnosis for this patient seems fairly obvious without the ENG, many patients who have severe vertigo at the time of their ENG examination frequently present problems both in the mechanics of testing and in their interpretation. In this instance there are both peripheral and central signs in the ENG, but I would personally be unwilling to place a probable site of lesion without a repeat examination in calmer circumstances.

We were able to confirm the clinically observed fine nystagmus in the primary eye position but beating in the opposite direction. The ENG does not confirm the clinical observation of a gaze nystagmus in all four gaze positions, only with upward gaze. There is no true gaze nystagmus in either lateral direction, but only a quite rapid oscillation without a quick and slow component (Fig. ENG-22-3). This, too, could be pathological, but the degree of motion is too small to attach much importance to it. The electrical (ENG) recording in such instances is probably more reliable than the average clinical observation for nystagmus. When eye movements are fine and rapid, it is difficult to distinguish quick and slow phases. Thus muscle tremors can be mistaken for nystagmus and vice versa.

The vertical nystagmus is a very rare phenomenon and is classically attributed to lesions of the midbrain tegmentum. It is always pathological and always an important clinical sign.

Her spontaneous nystagmus has a vestibular origin. Note the changes that occur in different head positions. There is also considerable blink artifact variability in these positions. The behavior of this nystagmus (direction-fixed, position-influenced) cannot be used with precision to decide if it is caused by a peripheral or central vestibular lesion. One can say, however, that there is a high likelihood for near-the-periphery involvement because the normal postural influences remain.

Interpretation of the caloric-induced nystagmus is largely an exercise in adding and subtracting vectors from the underlying spontaneous nystagmus while allowing a fudge factor for eye blinks. The interpretation of a severely depressed right labyrinth is based strictly on the very limited effect of stimulating this ear on the spontaneous nystagmus. Clinically, left-versus-right in acute-onset vertigo is a risky decision unless there are associated signs and symptoms. It is better to repeat the examination in a few weeks.

Note also that when the rapid right-beating spontaneous nystagmus is suppressed by the left-warm caloric, large semiregular saccades appear rather than a smooth baseline. This is normal and quite commonly seen during suppression of a vestibular spontaneous nystagmus.

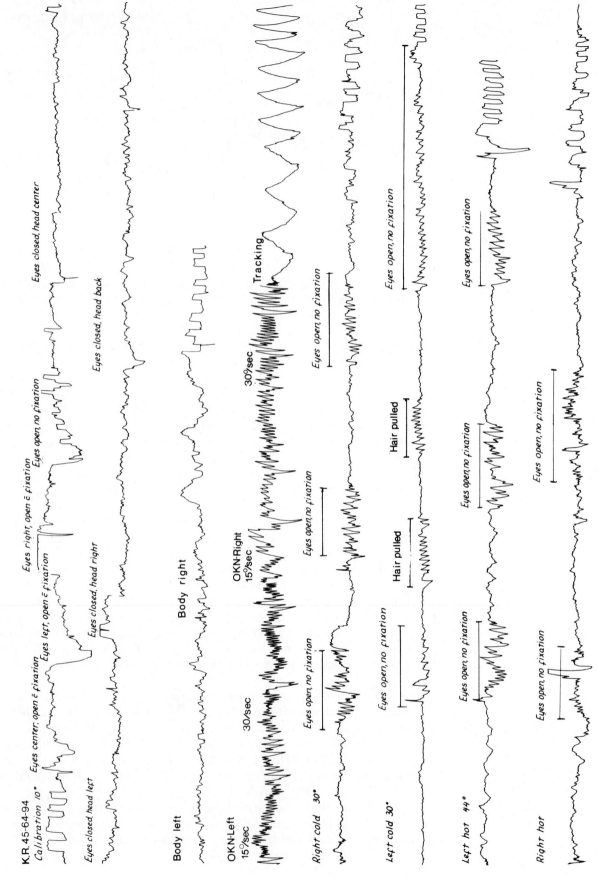

ENG-23.

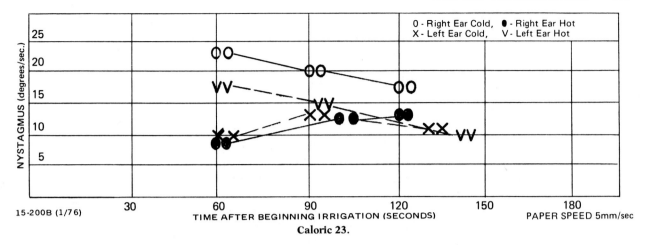

15-200B (1/7 6)

TIME AFTER BEGINNING IRRIGATION (SECONDS)

PAPER SPEED 5mm/sec

Caloric 23.

ENG-23

History: A 25-year-old female suffered a mild concussion in an automobile accident nearly a year ago. She feels dizzy all the time since the accident and has had four episodes of vomiting. She has a profound congenital hearing loss.

Examination is normal. There are no abnormal neurological signs. Audiogram shows profound sensorineural hearing loss in both ears, and an SRT could not be determined. Upon Lombard testing, the patient's voice became louder as the test noise became louder, thus indicating some exaggeration of the hearing loss. She also had some difficulty cooperating with the ENG test procedure.

ENG Report: There is no gaze, spontaneous, or position-induced nystagmus. Optokinetic nystagmus is symmetrical. There is essentially no caloric-induced nystagmus when tested in the standard manner with the eyes closed. Nystagmus was present with the eyes open. Such an effect can be pathological, but the same effect was also produced by a mild painful stimulus (hair pulling). Thus the decreased nystagmus was probably obtained on the basis of poor patient arousal. The caloric responses on the graph were obtained from the eyes-open segments.

Comments: This patient had moderate difficulty cooperating with the test procedure, and she performed poorly on alertness tasks. The present ENG shows a marked "FFS"; however, lightly pulling a few strands of hair (slight pain) also caused nystagmus to be accentuated. Thus the FFS present here is an artifact of poor patient arousal and should be ignored. A high index of suspicion is necessary to separate true FFS from arousal phenomena.

Although this ENG is reasonably explicable on the basis of an arousal problem, it does represent an extreme. Is this patient's degree of indifference to the test circumstances in itself normal or abnormal? I suspect it is abnormal. If my assumption is correct, the reason for the abnormality is equally obscure. This ENG has been included because it is an extreme level-of-arousal problem. It is a rare but dramatic example of the importance of this variable in testing patients.

Both Collins and Crampton and their co-workers have written extensively on the influence of arousal on both caloric and rotationally induced nystagmus.[12-14] Even in completely normal individuals, it is possible to manipulate this variable to cause changes in the slow-phase velocity of 300 percent and sometimes more. Contrast the possibilities for these large changes with the extreme care some ENG facilities take in ensuring 0.1°C accuracy in the temperature of the irrigating water—a variable of comparatively minor importance.

We have, for example, measured the effects of body temperature differences on calorics both during deliberate hyperthermia to 38.5°C and normally occurring variations of at least ±1°C. These persons, when stimulated with 30° and 44° irrigations, show no consistent or significant differences in nystagmus velocities from persons with normal body temperatures.

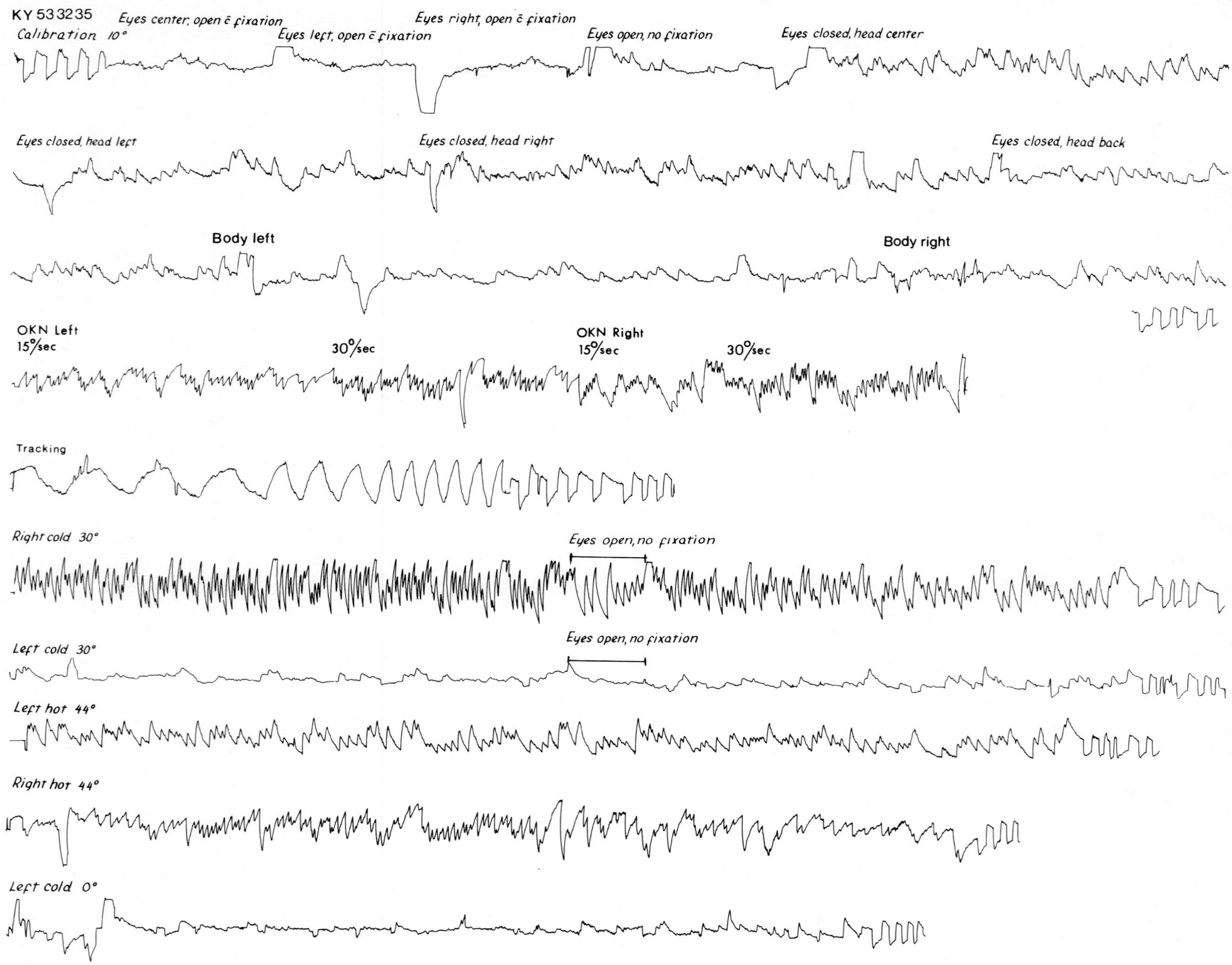

KY 53 3235

Calibration 10°

Eyes center, open c̄ fixation

Eyes right, open c̄ fixation

Eyes left, open c̄ fixation

Eyes closed, head center

Eyes open, no fixation

Eyes closed, head left

Eyes closed, head right

Eyes closed, head back

Body left

Body right

OKN Left
15°/sec

30°/sec

OKN Right
15°/sec

30°/sec

Tracking

Right cold 30°

Eyes open, no fixation

Left cold 30°

Eyes open, no fixation

Left hot 44°

Right hot 44°

Left cold 0°

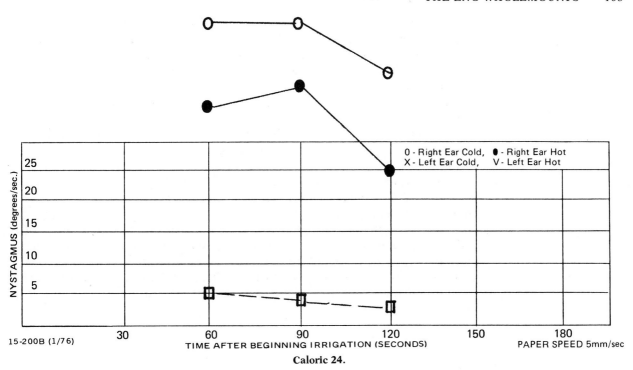

Caloric 24.

ENG-24

History: This 22-year-old male, a butcher, was lifting a heavy piece of meat 6 weeks before and heard a loud pop in his left ear. There was immediate tinnitus, vertigo, and hearing loss. An audiogram 4 weeks later showed a "flat-contoured" sensorineural hearing loss on the left averaging 70 dB. He is still bothered by vertigo, has trouble riding his bicycle, and cannot right himself while swimming. Physical examination is normal except for the eighth cranial nerve.

ENG Report: There is no gaze or position-induced nystagmus. There is a slight left-beating spontaneous nystagmus (eyes open, no fixation) which increases to an 8°–10° per second velocity with eyes closed. Head- and body-left positions attenuate this nystagmus, and the head-right position accentuates it slightly. OPN tracking is asymmetrical but probably normal.

The left caloric-induced nystagmus responses are severely hypoactive, perhaps completely nonresponding.

IMPRESSION. Abnormal examination, spontaneous nystagmus with positional effect, and hypoactive or nonresponsive left caloric responses.

Clinical Impression: Sudden hearing loss syndrome, probably membrane break.

Comment: This is a fairly straightforward ENG for a recent-onset peripheral vestibular lesion. The asymmetrical OPNs are probably caused by the underlying spontaneous vestibular nystagmus in this instance. Remember, however, that such interaction is not always true. Spontaneous nystagmus and symmetrical or asymmetrical OPNs can co-exist as pathological findings.

The major reason for including this ENG is that the electrodes have been applied backwards. The clues are in the OPN and caloric tracings, and perhaps in gaze testing. An experienced technician would have recognized this, and it can happen. Part of the reader's responsibility is to check for even this simple type of artifact.

In my experience, nystagmus to caloric stimulation *never* beats in the wrong direction, although such "perverted nystagmus" has been described by others. I doubt that a "wrong-direction" nystagmus actually existed in those instances. It is far more likely that the tactile stimulus of the caloric caused enhancement of an otherwise subliminal spontaneous nystagmus that happened to be beating in the direction opposite to that of the expected caloric nystagmus.

Incidentally, complete loss of caloric function in sudden idiopathic hearing loss is uncommon and distinctly rare in patients with flat-contoured audiograms.[29]

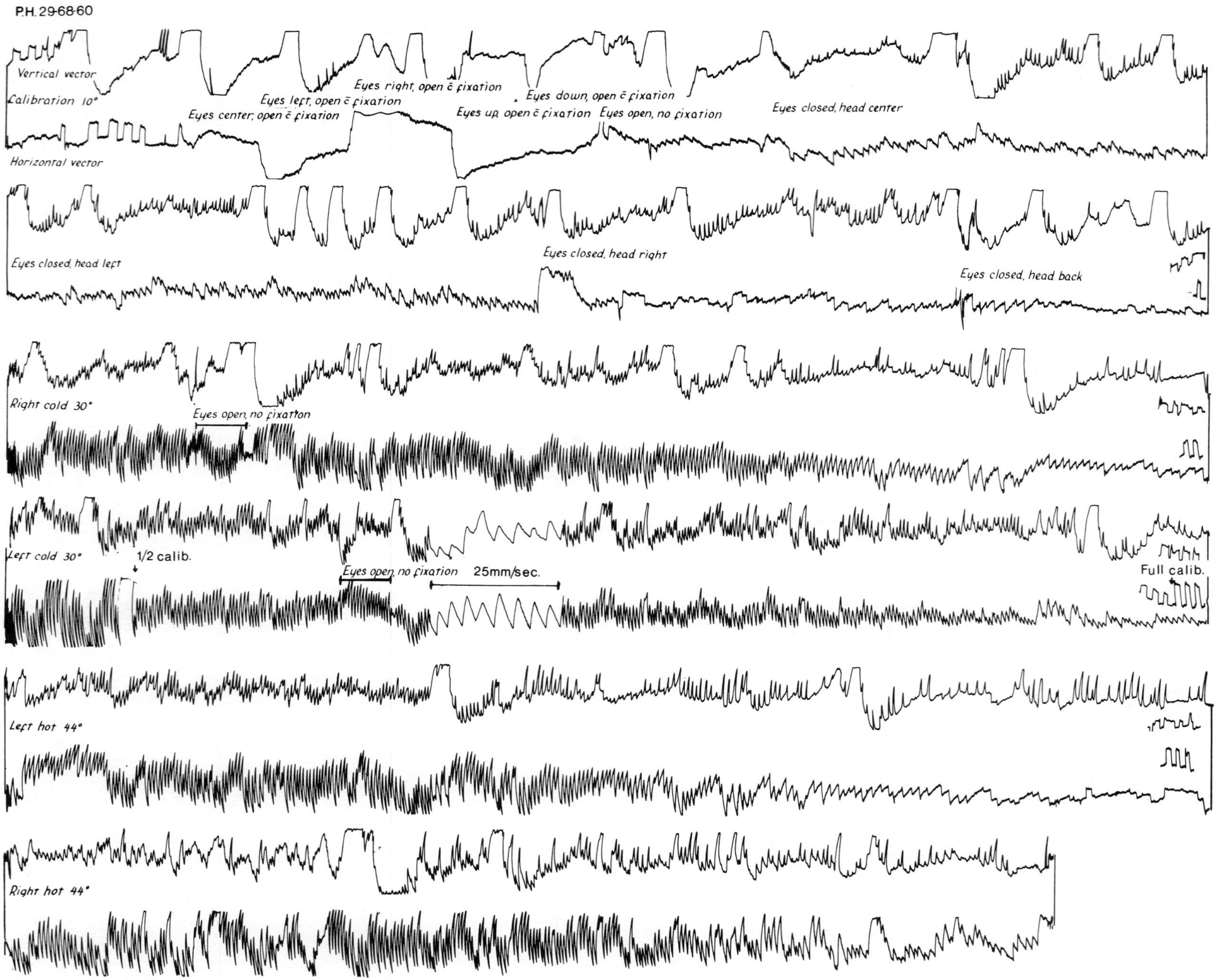

PH.29-6860

Vertical vector

Calibration 10°

Horizontal vector

Eyes center, open c̄ fixation

Eyes left, open c̄ fixation

Eyes right, open c̄ fixation

Eyes up open c̄ fixation

Eyes down, open c̄ fixation

Eyes open c̄ fixation

Eyes closed, head center

Eyes open, no fixation

Eyes closed, head left

Eyes closed, head right

Eyes closed, head back

Right cold 30°

Eyes open, no fixation

Left cold 30°

1/2 calib.

Eyes open, no fixation

25mm/sec.

Full calib.

Left hot 44°

Right hot 44°

ENG-25.

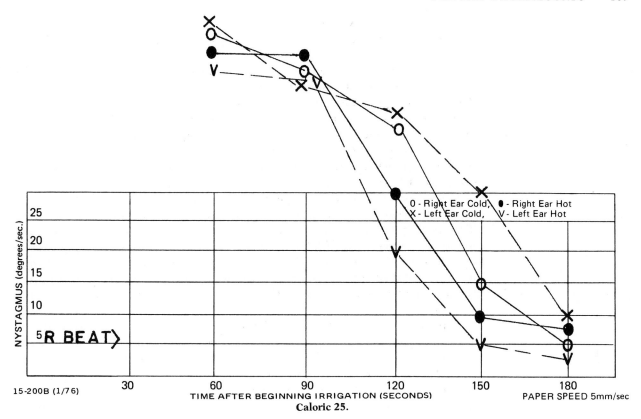

Caloric 25.

15-200B (1/76)

TIME AFTER BEGINNING IRRIGATION (SECONDS)

PAPER SPEED 5mm/sec

ENG-25

History: This 19-year-old female has a 1-month history of nystagmus and a 2-week history of oscillopsia, headaches with nausea, vomiting, and true vertigo with rapid head movements. She has a long history of migraine headaches and takes oral contraceptives. Examination shows a direction-changing spontaneous nystagmus, which is increased with head rotation, and an unsteady gait. Workup, including audiogram, brain scan, lumbar puncture, and vertebral arteriogram, was negative.

FOLLOW-UP. Pneumoencephalogram showed an ill-defined border of the left lateral recess of the fourth ventricle, suspicious for a left-cerebellar lesion but not confirmed. The patient was known to be pregnant 6 months later.

ENG Report: There is no gaze nystagmus. There is a right-beating spontaneous nystagmus when the eyes are open (no fixation). This nystagmus increases when the eyes are closed (approximate rate, 5°–8° per second) and is affected by head position: increased with head-left position and changing to a left-beating nystagmus with head-right position.
Bithermal caloric-induced nystagmus is symmetrical but hyperactive.

IMPRESSION. Abnormal examination, spontaneous nystagmus that changes direction in the head-right position, and hyperactive caloric nystagmus.

Comment: The ENG did not confirm the clinical observation of a direction-changing spontaneous nystagmus. The tracings show a spontaneous nystagmus that changes direction with head position—a position-induced, direction-changing nystagmus. There is an important diagnostic difference between these two types of nystagmus. A nystagmus that changes direction spontaneously is always pathological and always within the central nervous system. A position-related, direction-changing type is usually of central origin (about 70 percent) but can be peripheral, especially shortly after the onset of symptoms.

This woman received a very extensive neurological workup primarily because of her symptoms of oscillopsia in conjunction with vertigo and visual blurring. True oscillopsia (apparent transient oscillation of the visual field on sudden head motion or jarring, which lasts for a few tenths of a second) is almost always associated with complete or near-complete loss of functional otoliths or, if these are intact, of their central connections in the paleocerebellum. In this instance, it was quite unlikely that end-organ damage was present, because she has hyperactive calorics.

Hyperactive calorics are typically the result of heightened patient arousal (nervousness), and there are usually other signs of heightened arousal on the ENG, such as increased saccades, muscle tremor, and random baseline swings. These are not present in this ENG. Hyperactive calorics can also rarely be caused by midline posterior fossa lesions, and this is consistent with the patient's symptoms of oscillopsia.[18, 42]

Long-term Follow-up: Eight years later, the patient is still having balance problems, diplopia, and nystagmus. With this long history, a mass lesion seems highly unlikely. Oscillopsia is generally a grave sign, and the patient course makes one suspicious of the original diagnosis. The neurologist suspects a demyelinating disease.

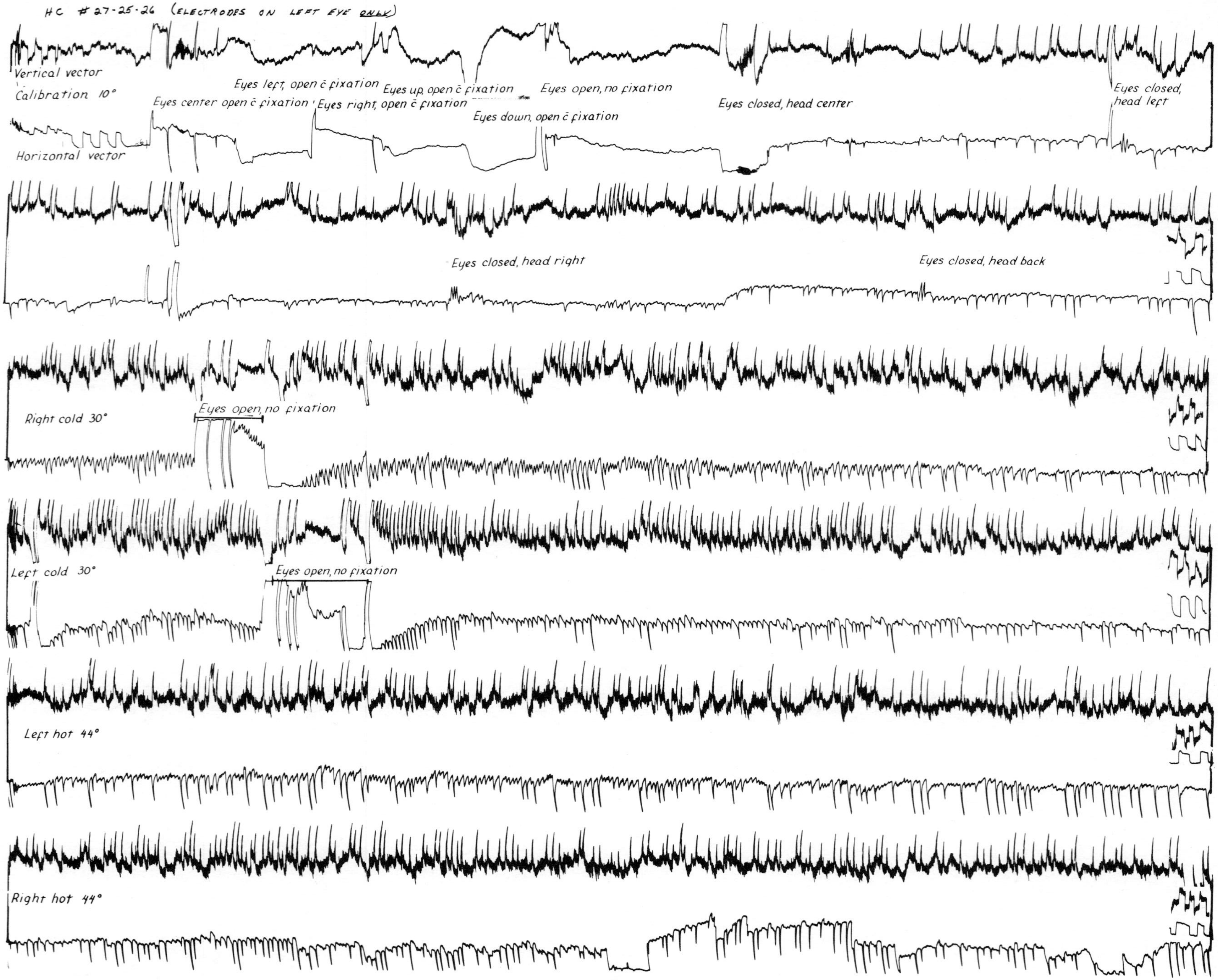

HC #27-25-26 (ELECTRODES ON LEFT EYE ONLY)

Vertical vector
Calibration 10°

Horizontal vector

Eyes left, open c̄ fixation   Eyes open, no fixation
Eyes center open c̄ fixation   Eyes right, open c̄ fixation
                              Eyes down, open c̄ fixation
Eyes up, open c̄ fixation

Eyes closed,
head left

Eyes closed, head back

Eyes closed, head center

Eyes closed, head right

Eyes open no fixation

Right cold 30°

Eyes open, no fixation

Left cold 30°

Left hot 44°

Right hot 44°

ENG-26.

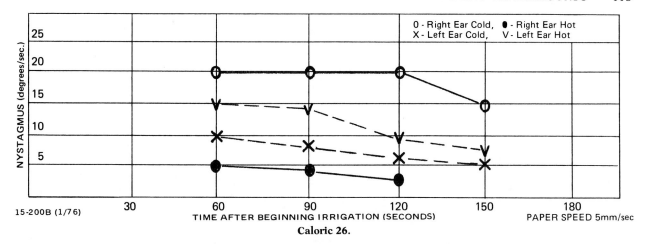

15-200B (1/76)

TIME AFTER BEGINNING IRRIGATION (SECONDS)

PAPER SPEED 5mm/sec

Caloric 26.

ENG-26

History: A 64-year-old female presents with a 6-week history of tinnitus and dizziness following an upper respiratory infection and a right ear discharge. Symptoms are aggravated by head or body motion and are brief and irregular. She has a past history of two strokes, 7 and 9 years ago; alleged "congenital atrophy of the right cerebral hemisphere"; and removal of the right eye for unknown cause. She has taken many oral medications for alleged Parkinson's disease. Examination shows a normal-appearing left eye, scarring on both tympanic membranes, and a left-beating nystagmus with left lateral gaze. There is a mild bilateral mixed hearing loss with normal discrimination and tone decay and no recruitment.

ENG Report: All recording is done on the left eye, her only eye. There is a consistent seeming inability for this patient to gaze rapidly toward the left, which can be noted especially in the irregular slope of the calibrations to the left. There does not appear to be any gaze nystagmus (contrary to clinical reports). When the patient's eye is closed, it deviates tonically upward and to the left (see Comment).

There is a slight and very fine left-beating nystagmus present when the lids are closed. This nystagmus is accentuated in the head-right position.

Bithermal caloric-induced nystagmus is asymmetrical, showing a nystagmus preponderance to the left, which is definitely outside the range of normal variation.

IMPRESSION. Abnormal examination, unusual eye motion (the left, her only eye) most suggestive of a muscle palsy, a spontaneous nystagmus that is affected by head position, and nystagmus preponderance of calorics toward the left.

Diagnosis: Probable vertebral-basilar artery disease, without confirmed anatomic diagnosis.

tal vector

Fig. ENG-26-1. Horizontal electrodes during calibration.

Comment: The calibration tracings are abnormal when the eye is deviated to the left (Fig. ENG-26-1). The rounding of the tracing suggests that pure lateral eye motion is not occurring and what is recorded is a vector from another plane of motion, most likely caused by an extraocular muscle palsy. The differential diagnosis of this calibration abnormality includes an unknown loss of one eye, an amblyopic eye, basal ganglion disease, extraocular muscle paralysis, and any other cause for discongruate eye motion.[45] There is no way to detect these defects per se from ENG; however, it is an important possibility if an ENG looks "peculiar."

Thus the "clinical impression" of a muscle palsy is not at all secure. Note that the fast phase nystagmus to the left during caloric stimulations is sharp and precise. A muscle paralysis is constant in its effect on eye motion. A good clinical observation would have eliminated (perhaps) such conjectures as to cause for a clearly abnormal left-tracking calibration tracing. OPN testing should have been done.

There is tonic deviation of the eye to the left which is consistently present even during caloric stimulation. The deviation is revealed specifically by deviation of the eyes to the left when the eyes are closed (see eyes-closed, head-center test) and apparent deviation to the right when the eyes are opened during calorics. The calorics show marked left directional preponderance which is consistent with left-sided tonic deviation.

The vertical tracing also exhibits 60-cycle background interference, which causes a uniform thickening of the baseline. This differs from an irregular thickening of the baseline caused by muscle noise (see ENG-17).

Many of the nystagmus beats are accentuated at their apex by a superimposed eyeblink, and these peaks should be disregarded in the measurement of the nystagmus velocity (see ENG-4).

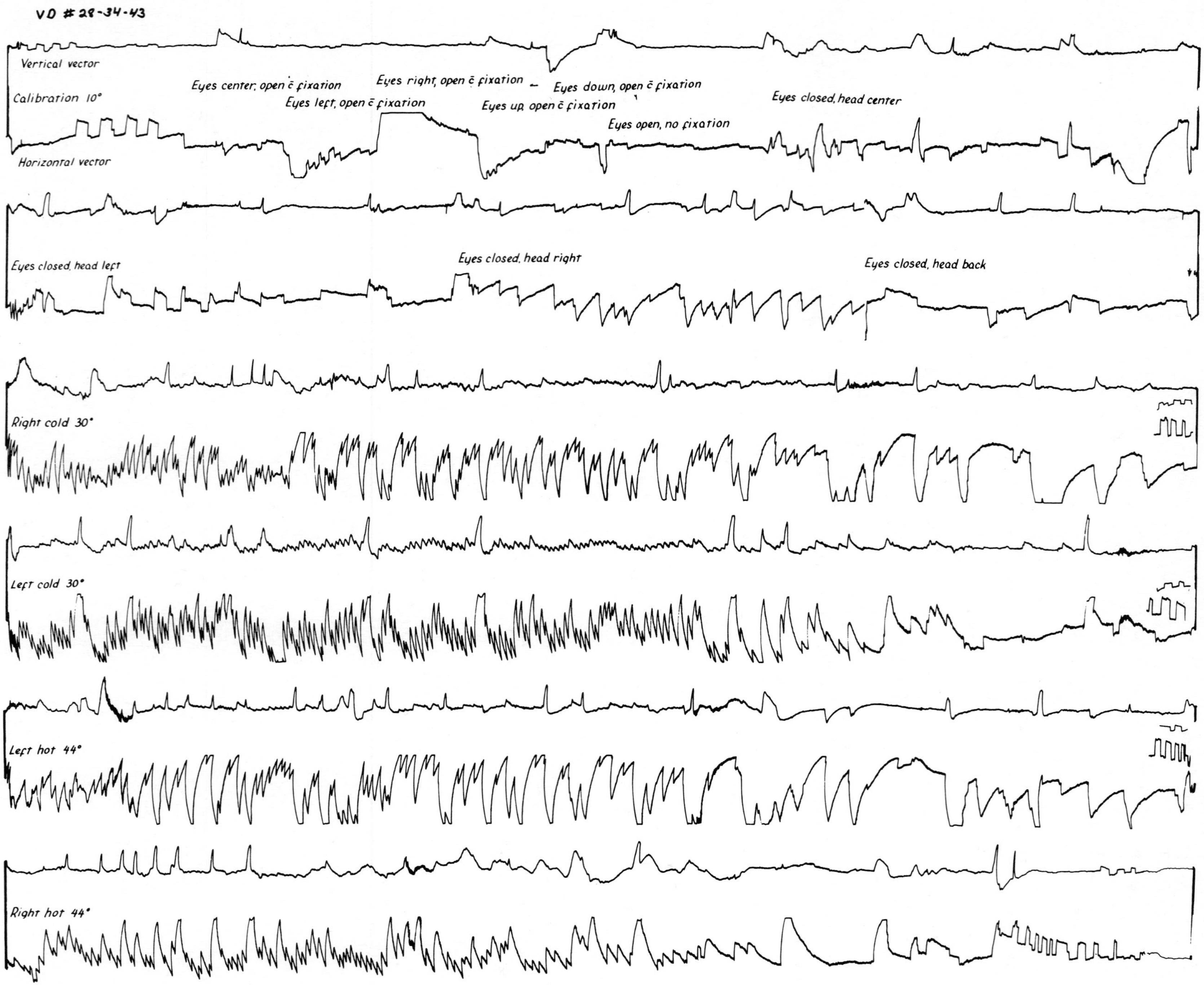

VD # 28-34-43

Vertical vector

Calibration 10°

Horizontal vector

Eyes center, open c̄ fixation   Eyes right, open c̄ fixation —   Eyes down, open c̄ fixation   Eyes closed, head center

Eyes left, open c̄ fixation   Eyes up open c̄ fixation

Eyes open, no fixation

Eyes closed, head left   Eyes closed, head right   Eyes closed, head back

Right cold 30°

Left cold 30°

Left hot 44°

Right hot 44°

ENG-27.

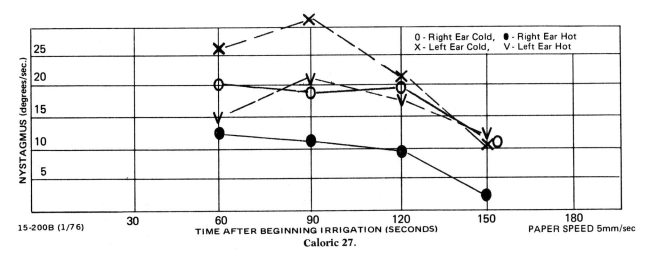

15-200B (1/76)

NYSTAGMUS (degrees/sec.)

TIME AFTER BEGINNING IRRIGATION (SECONDS)

PAPER SPEED 5mm/sec

Caloric 27.

0 - Right Ear Cold, ● - Right Ear Hot
X - Left Ear Cold, V - Left Ear Hot

ENG-27

History: This 53-year-old female had a sudden onset of vertigo and left tinnitus following a cervical hyperflexion-extension injury with retrograde amnesia secondary to an automobile accident. Examination shows "dizziness" with upward gaze. Audiometry 1 month after the accident shows an asymptomatic bilateral flat 20-dB sensorineural hearing loss.

ENG Report: There is both right and left lateral gaze nystagmus, but it is much more prominent to the left. There is a very coarse left-beating nystagmus in the head-right position (a coarseness more typical for cerebellar or CNS-induced nystagmus than labyrinthine nystagmus but not diagnostic thereof).

Bithermal caloric-induced nystagmus is asymmetrical and abnormal. While both left and right calorics have velocities within normal limits, the right responses are slower than those of the left. In addition, there is a dysmetria of the nystagmus beats, particularly when beating to the left.

IMPRESSION. Abnormal examination; gaze and positional nystagmus with asymmetrical and dysmetric calorics.

Follow-up: The patient was placed in a cervical collar and given symptomatic treatment; subsequent course indicated gradual improvement.

Comment: The fairly coarse gaze nystagmus and caloric dysmetria, coupled with a clinical history of amnesia and sudden neck trauma, strongly suggest that this woman also probably suffered cerebellar or brain stem injuries during her accident.

There was no clinical history available at the time of this ENG. Otherwise, the positional testing would also have been performed without neck torsion to check on the possibility that her positional nystagmus might have been secondary to neck motion. A test for visual suppression of the caloric nystagmus was not performed. It should have been.

IMPORTANT.   Dysmetria of caloric-induced nystagmus is a fairly rare finding and, in isolation from other findings, is a "soft" CNS sign without much localizing value. It is also a highly subjective observation by the ENG reader. Minor fluctuations in the nystagmus patterns should not be counted, and fluctuations in the patient's level of arousal as the cause should always be suspected and actively ruled out first. In this example, we cannot be absolutely certain about an arousal effect, except for the dominance of the dysmetria on left-beating nystagmus and the technician's confidence that this patient was adequately alerted throughout.

NOTE.   Calibrations of the vertical-vector electrodes for 10° of eye motion yielded only about 4 mm of pen deflection. This is not unusual and is a real problem with these electrodes. One solution, placing the electrodes nearer the orbit, usually only causes more muscle noise artifact.

There seems to be no consistent constellation of ENG abnormalities in patients with whiplash injuries and spatial disorientation. Ruben states that 50 percent have an ENG abnormality, most often positional nystagmus, typically to the same side as the neck injury. He has also observed reduced caloric responses on that same side.[38] Woods and Compere observed either a positional nystagmus or a spontaneous nystagmus influenced by head position.[46] My experience has been that spontaneous or positional nystagmus per se in persons with whiplash injuries is not very helpful, since the nystagmus velocities involved come very close to the boundary of normals. I feel more comfortable with patients such as this one, in whom there are also "soft" central nervous system signs, possibly indicating contusion. While I do perform the body rotation tests to check on the influence of neck torsion in patients with positional nystagmus, I have not been impressed with the results. I tend to agree with Coats, who said, "In some 5000 consecutive patients, I have not found a significant difference between nystagmus in the lateral neck-twisted and neck-straight positions."[10] Jonkees has written an excellent article on cervical vertigo.[25]

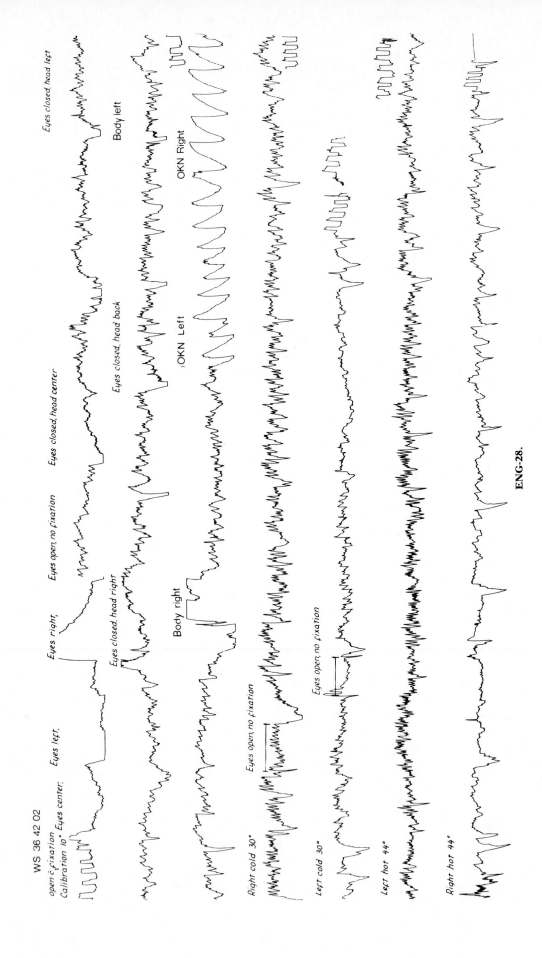

WS 36 42 02

open č fixation   Eyes left,   Eyes right,   Eyes open, no fixation   Eyes closed, head center   Eyes closed head left

Calibration 10° Eyes center,

Eyes closed, head right   Eyes closed, head back   Body left

Body right   OKN Left   OKN Right

Right cold 30°   Eyes open, no fixation

Left cold 30°   Eyes open, no fixation

Left hot 44°

Right hot 44°

ENG-28.

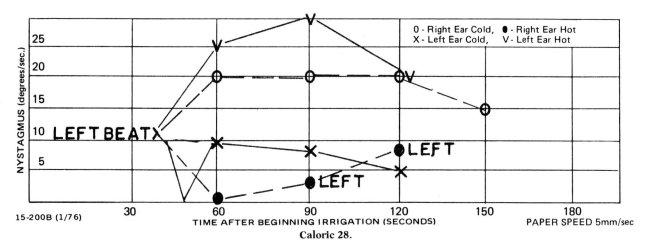

Caloric 28.

ENG-28

History: A 34-year-old male was seen 10 days after the insidious onset of an episodic sensation of disequilibrium lasting a few seconds. Four days ago, he noted the onset of acute "blockage" of his right ear and high-pitched tinnitus. Except for the hearing loss, there were no focal neurological symptoms.

His physical exam is normal. The audiogram shows a severe sensorineural loss in the right ear with an SRT of 90 dB and a discrimination of 20 percent. Internal auditory canal tomograms are normal.

ENG Report: There is no gaze nystagmus. There is a left-beating spontaneous nystagmus present with the eyes open (no fixation) at a rate of 7°–10° per second, which increases to a variable 10°–15° per second with the eyes closed. This nystagmus is increased with head-right and head-back positions and possibly also in the body-right position. Optokinetic nystagmus is symmetrical.

Bithermal caloric-induced nystagmus is asymmetrical. There is a comparatively hypoactive right ear and also a left nystagmus preponderance.

IMPRESSION. Abnormal examination, spontaneous nystagmus affected by head position, and asymmetrical caloric responses (see above).

Diagnosis: Sudden sensorineural hearing loss, cause unknown. His hearing improved to near-normal levels within 1 month.

Comment: This is a classic end-organ history and findings with one exception—the nystagmus seen with the eyes open did not increase spectacularly when the lids were closed. One would have expected at least a threefold increase.

This patient's nystagmus preponderance to the left with caloric stimulation is quite probably related to or created by his spontaneous nystagmus. Note, for

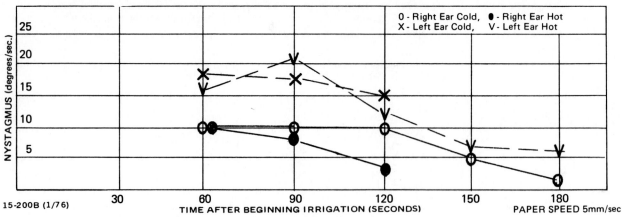

Fig. ENG-28-1. Caloric responses "corrected" for effect of spontaneous nystagmus (see text).

example, that the right-warm irrigation produces only enough of a response to suppress the left-beating spontaneous nystagmus and never does cause the normally expected right-beating nystagmus. Figure ENG-28-1 shows the calorics replotted with the spontaneous nystagmus vector subtracted—10° subtracted from the left-beating responses and 10° added to the right-beating responses. This "correction" now shows a hypoactive right ear, a finding that is consistent with the clinical facts of this patient.

Some ENG clinicians routinely "correct" caloric responses for spontaneous nystagmus on the assumption that there is always a relationship of the type hypothesized in this patient. I do not. There are no clear ground rules for determining the effect of a spontaneous nystagmus on the caloric responses. There are many times when it seems obvious on clinical grounds that caloric responses are not influenced by an underlying spontaneous nystagmus.

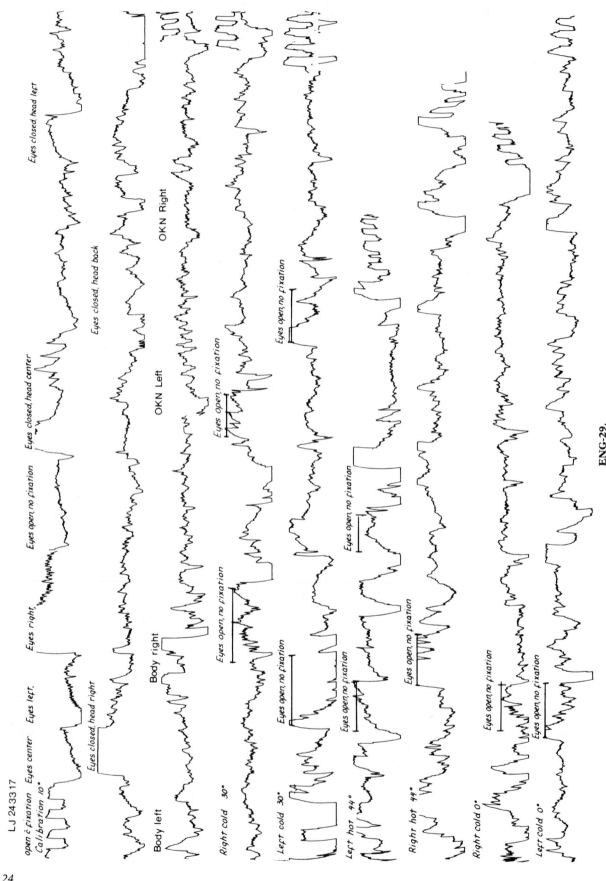

LJ 243317

Calibration 10°

open c̄ fixation   Eyes center   Eyes left,   Eyes right,   Eyes open, no fixation   Eyes closed, head center   Eyes closed head left

Eyes left,   Eyes closed, head right

Body left   Body right   Eyes closed, head back   OKN Right

OKN Left

Right cold 30°   Eyes open, no fixation   Eyes open, no fixation

Left cold 30°   Eyes open, no fixation   Eyes open, no fixation

Left hot 44°   Eyes open, no fixation   Eyes open, no fixation

Right hot 44°   Eyes open, no fixation

Right cold 0°   Eyes open, no fixation

Left cold 0°   Eyes open, no fixation

ENG-29.

124

ENG-29

History: A 42-year-old female with a long history of neurotic depression and a seizure disorder has a 10-year history of dizziness. She cannot identify predisposing or associated factors, except that they are posturally related and seem to be getting worse. She has increased difficulty walking in the dark. Her seizures are controlled with small amounts of antiepileptic medications. Six days ago, she was admitted to the hospital with acute barbiturate intoxication (overdose). There have been similar previous episodes.

Examination shows her unable to walk with eyes closed; when she walks, she slaps her left foot in a peculiar way and needs her vision to orient her movements. Systematic neurological examinations, by several examiners, including cerebellar tests, are negative. Audiogram shows a symmetrical, mild, low-frequency hearing loss. Internal auditory tomograms show minimal widening on the right.

ADDENDUM HISTORY. This patient had an established (and deserved) diagnosis of paranoid schizophrenia. She was examined several times by neurologists without positive findings and was lost to follow-up 5 months after her second ENG.

ENG Report: This patient has a bilateral fine but marked gaze nystagmus. During positional testing, there is considerable irregularity in the positioning of her eyes (lids closed), and while it cannot be determined with any degree of certainty if there is a spontaneous direction-changing nystagmus in the head-center position, there probably is. Also, in the several other head and body positions, there appears to be nystagmus from time to time, always irregular and unsustained.

Optokinetic nystagmus testing is definitely abnormal. She tracks poorly and irregularly in both lateral directions.

There is only a minimal response to bithermal caloric stimuli and to ice water stimulation. Nystagmus is only observed with the eyes open except for a brief early period during ice water stimulation of the right ear.

IMPRESSION. Abnormal examination, gaze nystagmus, questionable spontaneous direction-changing nystagmus, poor optokinetic tracking, and severely depressed caloric responses that demonstrate absence of normal visual suppression.

COMMENT. If one did not know this patient's recent drug history, one would presume that a severe central nervous system abnormality is present. This test should be repeated when we can be certain, very certain, that no sedatives or related drugs, including diphenylhydantoin and antihistamines, have been ingested for at least 72 hours.

NOTE. A follow-up ENG was performed 6 weeks later. The gaze nystagmus (but not the tremor) and spontaneous nystagmus were no longer present. OPN and caloric results were essentially unchanged.

Comment: Diphenylhydantoin, at blood level concentrations exceeding 15 mg/100 ml, is the most common drug-induced cause for weird ENGs that most typically mimic posterior fossa ENG abnormalities, including gaze nystagmus of the coarse variety.* Barbiturates typically have two effects, a direction-changing, position-induced nystagmus (similar to alcohol) and a more general alertness depression effect. Signs on an ENG can be present for as long as 10 days after ingestion.

In this ENG, there was probably a mixture of drug and nondrug abnormalities. Since the gaze and spontaneous nystagmus disappeared on the follow-up ENG, these were probably drug related. However, I am unaware of any drug correlations with a spontaneous direction-changing nystagmus which seemed to be present here. Caloric-induced nystagmus is not radically affected by drugs unless the patient is severely obtunded (fast phase disappears). Thus the lack of caloric responses and also probably the OPN abnormality reflect anatomic lesions, site undetermined. My suspicions favor a posterior fossa or lower midbrain locale.

---

* Therapeutic range is generally 10–20 mg/100 ml.

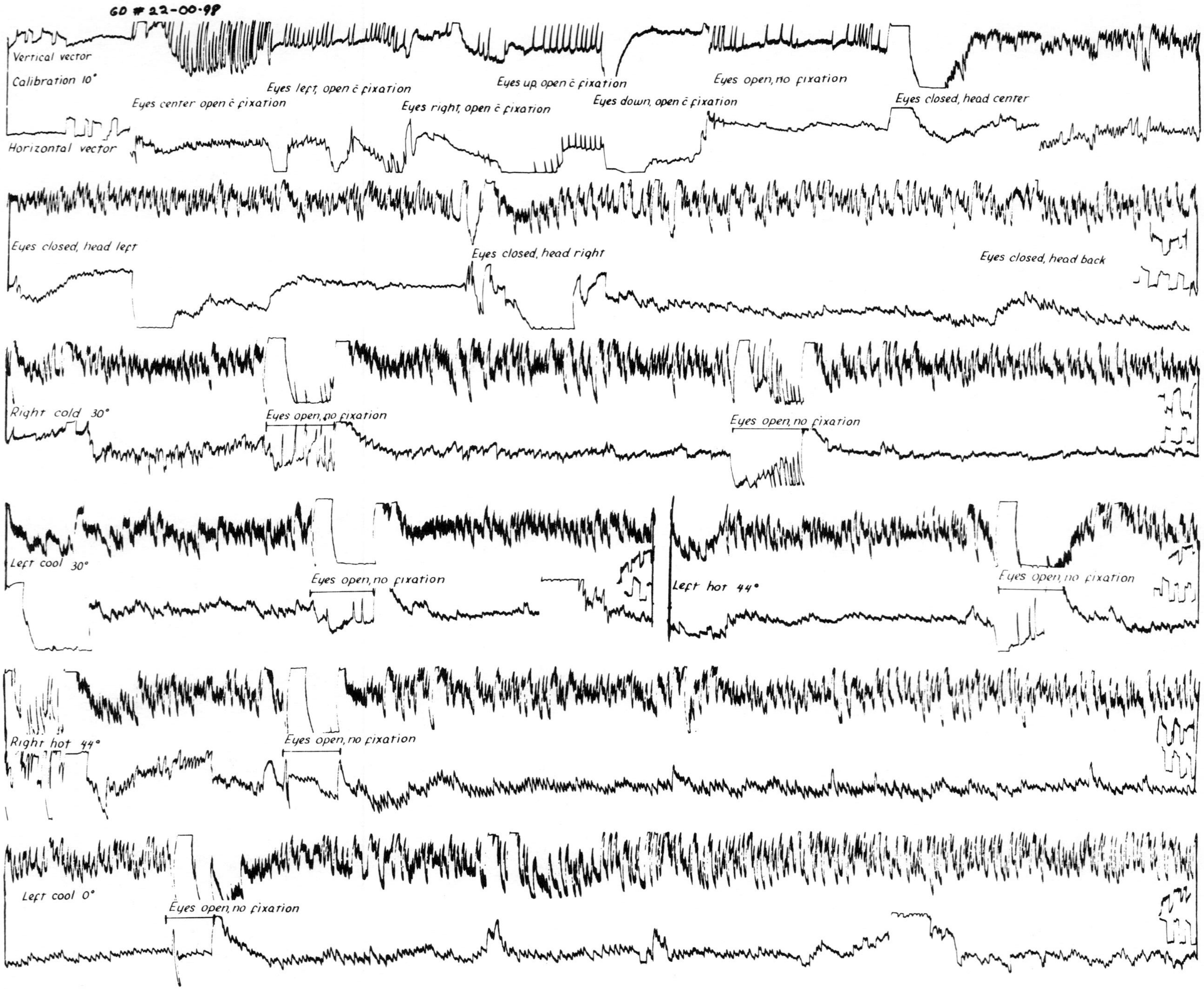

GO # 22-00-99

Vertical vector

Calibration 10°

Eyes center open ċ fixation

Eyes open, no fixation

Eyes closed, head center

Eyes up open ċ fixation

Eyes down, open ċ fixation

Eyes left, open ċ fixation

Eyes right, open ċ fixation

Horizontal vector

Eyes closed, head left

Eyes closed, head right

Eyes closed, head back

Right cold 30°

Eyes open, no fixation

Eyes open, no fixation

Left cool 30°

Eyes open, no fixation

Left hot 44°

Right hot 44°

Eyes open, no fixation

Eyes open, no fixation

Left cool 0°

Eyes open, no fixation

ENG-30.

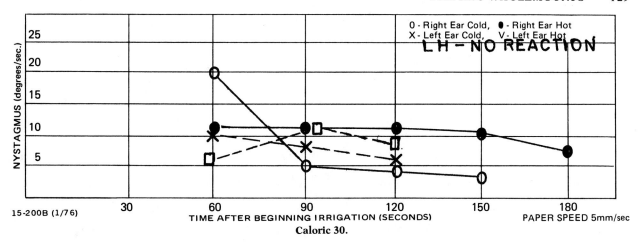

Caloric 30.

ENG-30

History: This 80-year-old male had a history of two 3-day episodes of vertigo and disequilibrium within the last 2 weeks. Three years previously, he had a basal cell carcinoma removed from his left cheek. Tumor was present at the margins of the specimen, and he subsequently had radiation therapy. Two years ago, he had a spontaneous left facial paralysis unaccompanied by other neurological symptoms or x-ray abnormality. The patient had no symptoms of dry eye and no alteration in taste. A neurosurgical consultant thought it represented an idiopathic facial paralysis (Bell's palsy). Five months ago, the patient developed a slight left hearing loss (end-organ type) that has progressed slightly.

Examination shows a complete facial paralysis and left serous otitis media. Audiogram shows moderate sensorineural hearing loss plus a 30-dB air-bone gap. X-ray studies show destruction of the left base of skull, the petrous pyramid, and the left internal auditory meatus. Granulation tissue removed from the middle ear via tympanotomy was negative for tumor.

ENG Report: There is a coarse left-gaze nystagmus with many interposed eye blinks. There is irregular abnormal random eye motion (not a nystagmus) present with fixation and with eyes closed, but this does not occur when the eyes are open without fixation. There is a right-beating positional nystagmus that is most marked in head-right and head-back positions. The vertical channel is technically unsatisfactory because of blinking and muscle movement noise.

Bithermal caloric-induced nystagmus responses are hypoactive on the right and probably absent on the left.

IMPRESSION.   Abnormal examination, coarse left gaze nystagmus, right-beating positional nystagmus, and abnormal caloric responses bilaterally.

Follow-up: Neurosurgical differential diagnosis included metastatic skin neoplasm or perhaps invasive acoustic neuroma or glomus jugulare. The patient was not thought to be a candidate for further workup, and he was given 5000 rads to the left base of the skull. Six months later, tomograms showed regression of the lytic changes in the petrous bone. The patient lived another 3 years and eventually died with local recurrence of tumor and probably cerebral abscess.

Comment: This is a complicated ENG, with several problems in interpretation. First, there appears to be a spontaneous right-beating nystagmus. Is this visual or vestibular in origin? This nystagmus is present with visual fixation but disappears when fixation is prevented and then reappears with the eyes closed (head-center position). If this were truly a visual system nystagmus, it ought to diminish (or disappear) when fixation is prevented and certainly not reappear when the eyes are closed. Also, if the nystagmus is truly fixation-related, it should be present during calibration trackings. It is not. On the other hand, if it is a vestibular nystagmus, it should increase when fixation is prevented and be much more marked with the eyes closed.

The "nystagmus" seen on this tracing conforms to neither of these patterns. In fact, on close inspection (see Fig. ENG-30-1), the eye motions are not truly nystagmoid at all but are quite rapid to-and-fro movements of the eyeball with neither fast nor slow component.

The next problem arises in interpreting the position-related nystagmus. There is a marked right-beating nystagmus in the head-right and head-back positions and which, with a little imagination, may also be present in the head-left position. One wonders if this is not truly an accentuation of a latent head-center spontaneous nystagmus because it persists during the caloric stimulation of the apparently nonfunctioning left labyrinth.

The vertical electrodes, as usual, do not help. They do show lots of electrical activity—lid flutter and eye blinks early in the tracing; perhaps a nystagmus once the lids are closed but mixed with lid flutter, 60-cycle artifact, and blinks; and then considerable muscle noise during the calorics.

The interpretation of caloric response in the presence of spontaneous nystagmus can be a difficult problem because one must differentiate between a true caloric response and an increase in the spontaneous nystagmus secondary to tactile stimulation. The first differentiating feature is the time of onset of response after stimulus. A normal caloric will have a delay of 30 to 40 seconds before a nystagmus starts, whereas a purely tactile stimulus will have an immediate incremental effect on the spontaneous nystagmus. Second, a caloric response should have a predictable pattern of slow-phase velocity, reaching a maximum at about 90

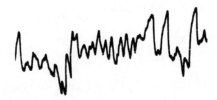

Fig. ENG-30-1. Segment of eyes-closed, head-center tracing at about 25 seconds.

seconds, and then decaying over the next 2 minutes or so. An arousal effect caused by tactile stimulation does not show this pattern.

There is a clear response to right-cool stimulation, since this beats toward the left and reverses the right-beating background nystagmus. The right-warm stimulus accentuates this right-beating nystagmus, as would be expected.

The nystagmus during left-cool stimulation is in the expected direction but does not exceed the range of the background nystagmus. This is confirmed by ice water irrigation of the left ear (bottom tracing) which produces an unimpressive accentuation of the right-beating nystagmus. There is no change in the pattern during left-warm stimulation. It would appear that there is very little, if any, response coming from the left ear, only an accentuation of the background nystagmus secondary to the tactile stimulation of water in the ear canal.

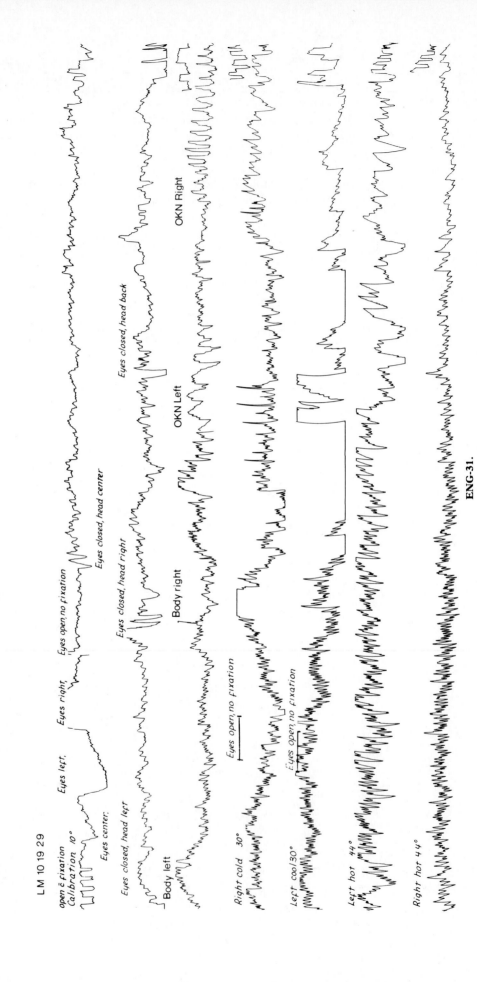

ENG-31.

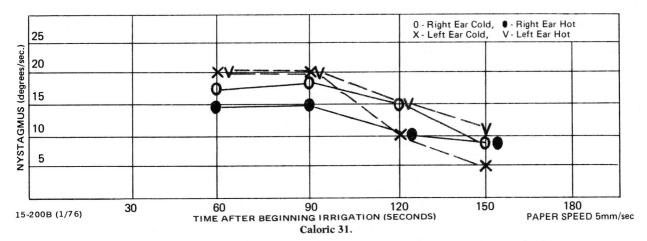

0 - Right Ear Cold,   ● - Right Ear Hot
X - Left Ear Cold,   V - Left Ear Hot

15-200B (1/76)

TIME AFTER BEGINNING IRRIGATION (SECONDS)

PAPER SPEED 5mm/sec

Caloric 31.

ENG-31

History: This 57-year-old female experienced two episodes of true vertigo, lasting approximately 20 minutes each, 1 and 2 months ago. This occurred while changing from the supine to the upright position when she awoke in the morning. The vertigo passed spontaneously but left her with a sensation of minor disequilibrium. She is not aware of any hearing loss, tinnitus, fullness within the ears, otalgia, or any neurological symptom. She has suffered severe cervical arthritis that nearly required surgery but has responded to conservative management. Audiogram and neurological examination are normal.

ENG Report: There is no gaze nystagmus. An intermittent left-beating spontaneous nystagmus is present at the rate of 1°–3° per second. A direction-changing, position-induced nystagmus to the right in head-left position and to the left in head-right position is present. This nystagmus is increased with body rotation. Optokinetic tracking is abnormal in both directions.

   Bithermal caloric-induced nystagmus is within normal limits for nystagmus velocity and right-left symmetry.

   IMPRESSION.   Abnormal examination; spontaneous and direction-changing, position-induced nystagmus and abnormal OPN responses.

Comment: This ENG does not relate well to the patient's clinical history or to the negative physical findings. The slight spontaneous nystagmus is inconsequential. The position-induced, direction-changing nystagmus is most definitely pathological, especially as recorded in the body-turned positions. This woman vehemently denied taking any drugs, and if this is correct, the cause must be somewhere in the central nervous system. The bilateral OPN abnormality is clearly present at both speeds to the right and one to the left. Yet this patient had no other clinical findings, and on follow-up 4 years later, she was leading an uneventful life, having had only one further episode of vertigo.

The most common cause for bilaterally abnormal OPN is in the posterior fossa. Drugs can also cause bilateral problems. Coates analyzed 1228 consecutive ENGs and found that 7 percent had abnormal OPNs. Of these, 1 percent were caused by ocular abnormalities (mainly congenital); 1 percent were caused by a strong vestibular nystagmus inhibiting eye movement in one direction and enhancing it in the other; slightly over 2 percent were from central nervous system causes (typically posterior fossa); and 2 percent had no explanation.[9] This patient fits this last group rather well.

I suspect that the commonly held notion that OPN asymmetries and dysmetria are always pathological, in the clinically important sense of the word, does not hold for high-quality ENG recordings. Remember that nearly all the experience on OPN was obtained by direct visual inspection and using fairly crude OPN stimuli that are likely to demonstrate only large differences. ENG recordings are more sensitive and likely to yield more abnormals, some of which are not clinically important.

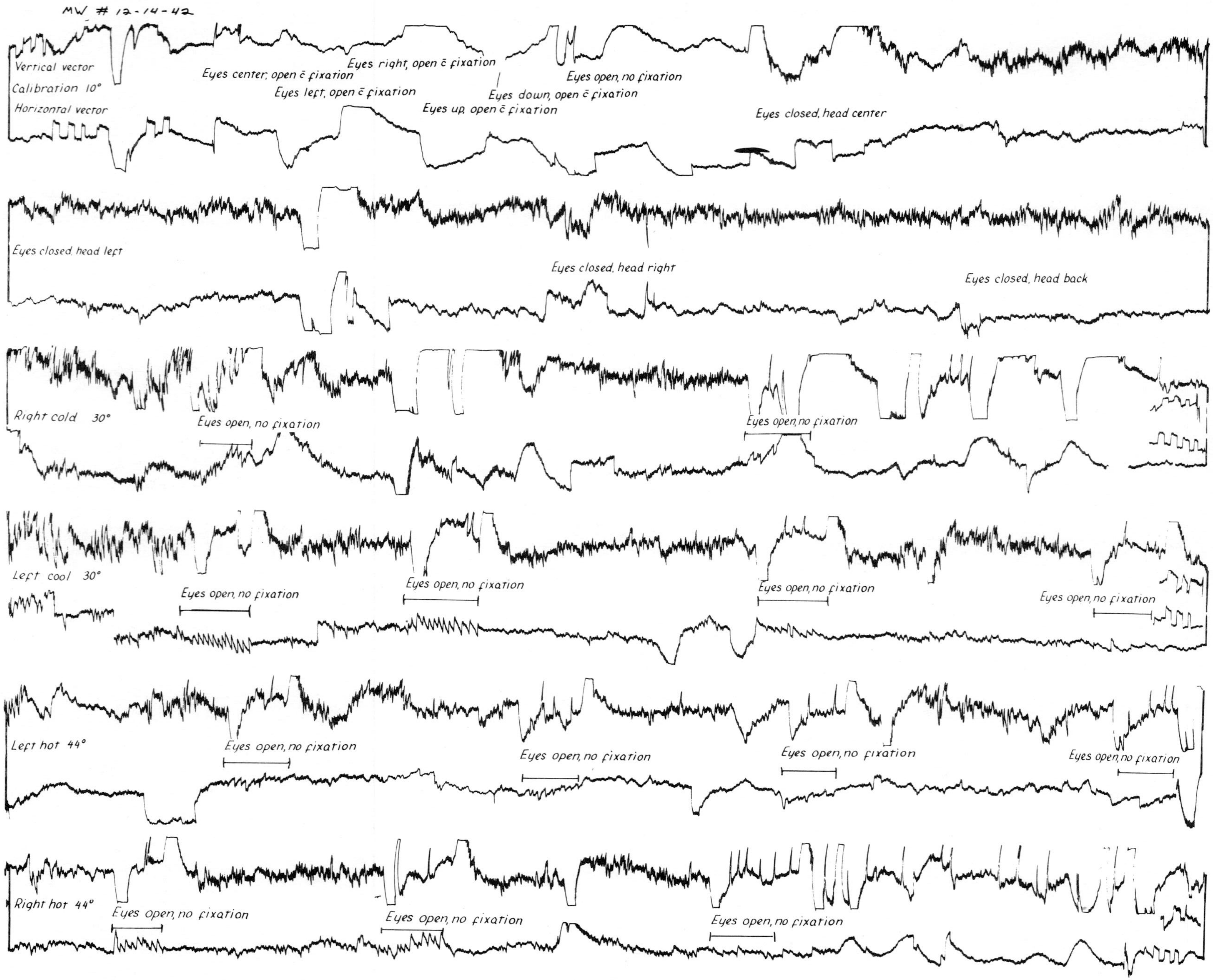

MV # 12-14-42

Vertical vector
Calibration 10°
Horizontal vector

Eyes center, open ē fixation
Eyes right, open ē fixation
Eyes left, open ē fixation
Eyes up, open ē fixation
Eyes down, open ē fixation
Eyes open, no fixation

Eyes closed, head center

Eyes closed head left

Right cold 30°

Eyes open, no fixation

Eyes open, no fixation

Eyes closed, head back

Eyes closed, head right

Eyes open, no fixation

Left cool 30°

Eyes open, no fixation

Eyes open, no fixation

Eyes open, no fixation

Left hot 44°

Eyes open, no fixation

Eyes open, no fixation

Eyes open, no fixation

Right hot 44°

Eyes open, no fixation

Eyes open, no fixation

ENG-32.

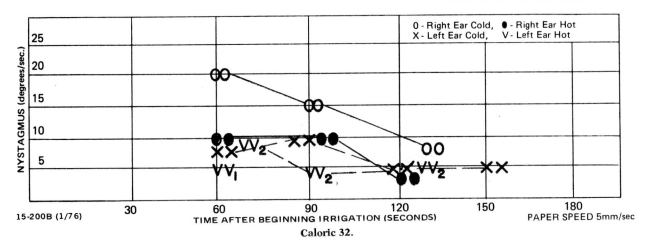

Caloric 32.

ENG-32

History: A 35-year-old male physician presents with episodic recurrent postural vertigo. The first episode, 3 years ago, was characterized by transient attacks of vertigo that occurred while he was changing from an erect to a supine position or vice versa, especially if his head was turned toward the right. At the same time, he also had some unsteadiness of gait. He was free of symptoms until recently, when he developed similar symptoms, particularly upon turning his head toward the right in the supine position. Five years ago the patient had an episode of "benign viral encephalopathy" characterized by headaches. Lumbar puncture and other examinations were all normal except for 80 mg/100 ml of protein.

ENG Report: There is no gaze, spontaneous, or position-induced nystagmus. Bithermal caloric-induced responses are most unusual. There is very little nystagmus observable when the lids are closed, but an almost normal amount when the eyes are open (fixation prevented). The left ear responses are hypoactive.

IMPRESSION. Abnormal examination, hypoactive left labyrinth to caloric stimulation, and unusual and possibly pathological CNS inversion of eyes-open, eyes-closed amounts of vestibular-induced nystagmus (failure of fixation suppression).

Diagnosis: Probably benign paroxysmal postural vertigo. On follow-up, he has had no further attacks.

Follow-up: According to the *Directory of Medical Specialists*, the patient was still in practice 8 years later.

Comment: The increase of nystagmus with the eyes open during caloric-induced nystagmus is a highly significant finding. There are three possible explanations:

1.   A CNS defect, location not specified, of visual-vestibular pathways.
2.   Depressed or severely altered level of arousal when lids are closed—sleepy, on medication, and so on.
3.   A tonic deviation of the eyes with lids closed. If the eyes are rotated upward with eyes closed, as in Bell's phenomenon, the horizontal electrodes may be incapable of detecting nystagmus. If, however, the eyes assume normal position when open, nystagmus is recorded. Evidence for his hypothesis may be found in the vertical tracing here. Note that when the eyes are opened there is a tonic change inposition downward and a return upward when the eyes are closed again. I would not personally rest easily with this explanation without a complete neurological clearance.

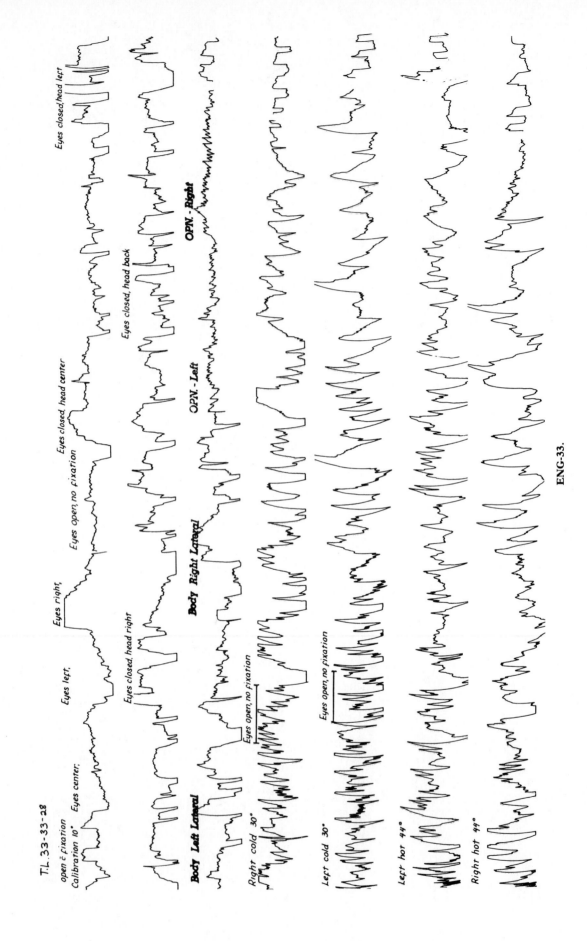

T.L. 33-33-28

open č fixation

Calibration 10°

Eyes center,

Eyes left,

Eyes right,

Eyes open, no fixation

Eyes closed, head center

Eyes closed, head left

Eyes closed, head right

Eyes closed, head back

Body Left Lateral

OPN - Left

OPN - Right

Right cold 30°

Eyes open, no fixation

Body Right Lateral

Left cold 30°

Eyes open, no fixation

Left hot 44°

Right hot 44°

ENG-33.

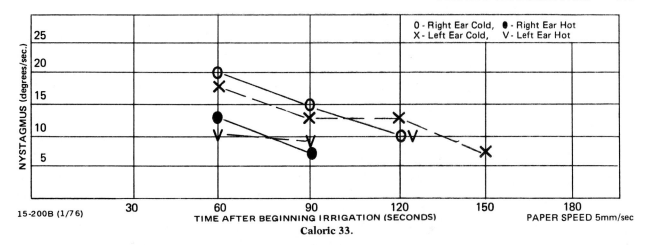

Caloric 33.

15-200B (1/76)

ENG-33

History: This 57-year-old male developed a right central facial weakness, ataxia, and right hemiparesis 3 weeks ago. He has biopsy-proven undifferentiated large cell carcinoma of the mediastinum which was irradiated 8 months ago. Ten years ago, the patient had a right cerebral vascular accident with a left-sided hemiparesis from which he recovered. Exam shows a right trigeminal hypoesthesia, right central facial weakness, positive Romberg, and past-pointing to the left. There was a right-sided hemiparesis and hypoesthesia of the extremities. There was a bilaterally equal, mild sensorineural hearing loss with no tone decay. Brain scan showed increased left frontal uptake.

ENG Report: There is irregular calibration tracking. The patient seems unable to maintain visual fixation on the calibration target for more than a few tenths of a second. There is no gaze, spontaneous, or position-induced nystagmus present with eyes open or closed. There are multiple wide swings of the pen during positional testing, suggestive of a loose electrode. OPN is asymmetrical and abnormal when tracking to the left.

Bithermal caloric-induced nystagmus is within normal limits for nystagmus velocity and right-left symmetry; however, there is a significant and symmetrical dysmetria present in all calorics.

IMPRESSION. Abnormal examination, OPN asymmetry, poor calibration tracking, and dysmetric caloric nystagmus; visual system disorder should be ruled out.

Diagnosis: Neurosurgeons elected to treat the patient with radiation therapy to the brain. He subsequently expired with cerebral metastases.

Comment: The calibration tracings are consistently poor and most likely indicate difficulty in seeing the target. A good place in the ENG to check on this is during OPN testing, since this visual stimulus is less dependent on good peripheral vision. Note here that the OPNs are also poorly formed, especially on left tracking. This might correlate with his left frontal brain scan abnormality if the right OPN were abnormal. However, there are too many alternative possibilities in the past history.[19] This patient was also taking sedatives, and these, too, can cause poor tracking performances.

Although there are no specifically identifiable vestibular or nystagmus abnormalities in this exam, the patient's general eye motion is extremely irregular and very coarse—responses that would be within normal limits for a 3- or 4-year-old child but not for an adult.

Responses to caloric stimulation are quite dysrhythmic. This may be the result of his medications (propoxyphene and diazepam) but probably is not and should be considered pathological until proven otherwise.

Be suspicious of a loose electrode when the pen swings all the way off the tracing from time to time, particularly when the velocity is high. Also note that in this tracing, nearly all of these swings are associated with head movement off the midplane. The underlying cause for the violent pen movement off the tracing is typically the large transient voltage received by the amplifier. The voltage is created by movement-induced changes in the skin-electrode interface. Even though this movement is transient, the induced voltage sometimes saturates the amplifier, and the pen will remain off the paper until this voltage is discharged. The rate of this discharge is controlled by the frequency response of ENG machines and will therefore be different depending on the machine. A machine with very good low-frequency sensitivity (long time constant) will require a longer period of time. A machine with very poor high-frequency sensitivity may never reveal loose electrode effects because the transient voltage surge will be filtered out within the amplifier. Thus, a machine with a limited frequency band pass will produce more even tracings but at a considerable sacrifice in accuracy.

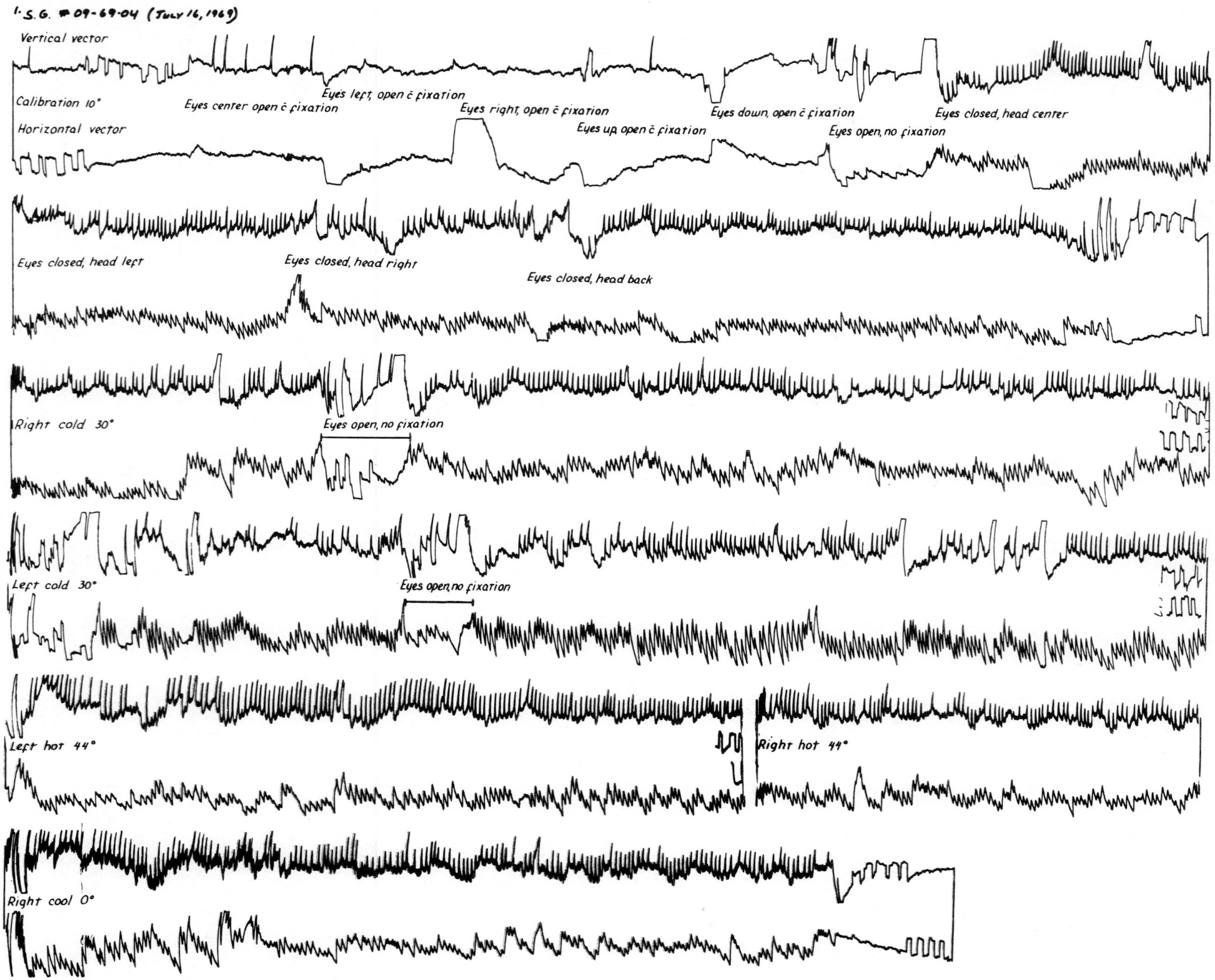

I. S. G. # 09-69-04 (Jan 16, 1969)

Vertical vector

Calibration 10°

Horizontal vector

Eyes center open ċ fixation

Eyes left, open ċ fixation

Eyes right, open ċ fixation

Eyes up open ċ fixation

Eyes down open ċ fixation

Eyes open, no fixation

Eyes closed, head center

Eyes closed, head left

Eyes closed, head right

Eyes closed, head back

Right cold 30°

Eyes open, no fixation

Left cold 30°

Eyes open, no fixation

Left hot 44°

Right hot 44°

Right cool 0°

ENG-34A.

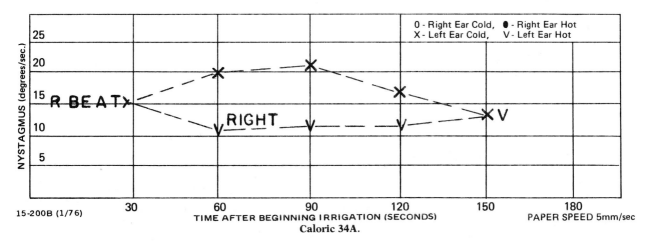

Caloric 34A.

ENG-34

History: A 22-year-old female presents with recent onset of constant tinnitus and fullness in the right ear and dizziness occurring two to three times a week. She had a severe cerebral injury in an auto accident 8 years ago, which required burr-hole craniotomy for left subdural hematoma. Examination shows a positive Romberg to the right. Audiogram shows a severe right low-frequency hearing loss with 54 percent discrimination and complete recruitment.

ENG Report 1: There is no gaze nystagmus. There is a right-beating spontaneous nystagmus with the eyes open and no fixation, and this is increased to >15° per second when the eyes are closed. There is no body position effect.

Bithermal caloric-induced nystagmus shows a normal response to stimulation with cold water in the left ear, a hypoactive response to stimulation with warm water in the left ear, and no response to any stimulation in the right.

IMPRESSION. Abnormal examination, spontaneous nystagmus unaffected by head position, hypoactive caloric response to left-warm stimulation, and no response to any stimulation in the right ear.

CLINICAL COMMENT. This patient is a none-too-reliable historian as a result of brain damage incurred in an auto accident at age 15 and has had balance problems since. She states her balance is not troubling her at this time, when it is, in fact, very poor on clinical observation. I have no way of knowing if the ENG findings are old or recent, but I suspect that the majority are long standing. We do, however, need a second exam in about 2 weeks to check this point.

ENG Report 2: This is a repeat examination for comparison with one obtained 3 weeks previously. There is a marked decrease in the patient's spontaneous nystagmus (a change from greater than 15° per second to about 5° per second).

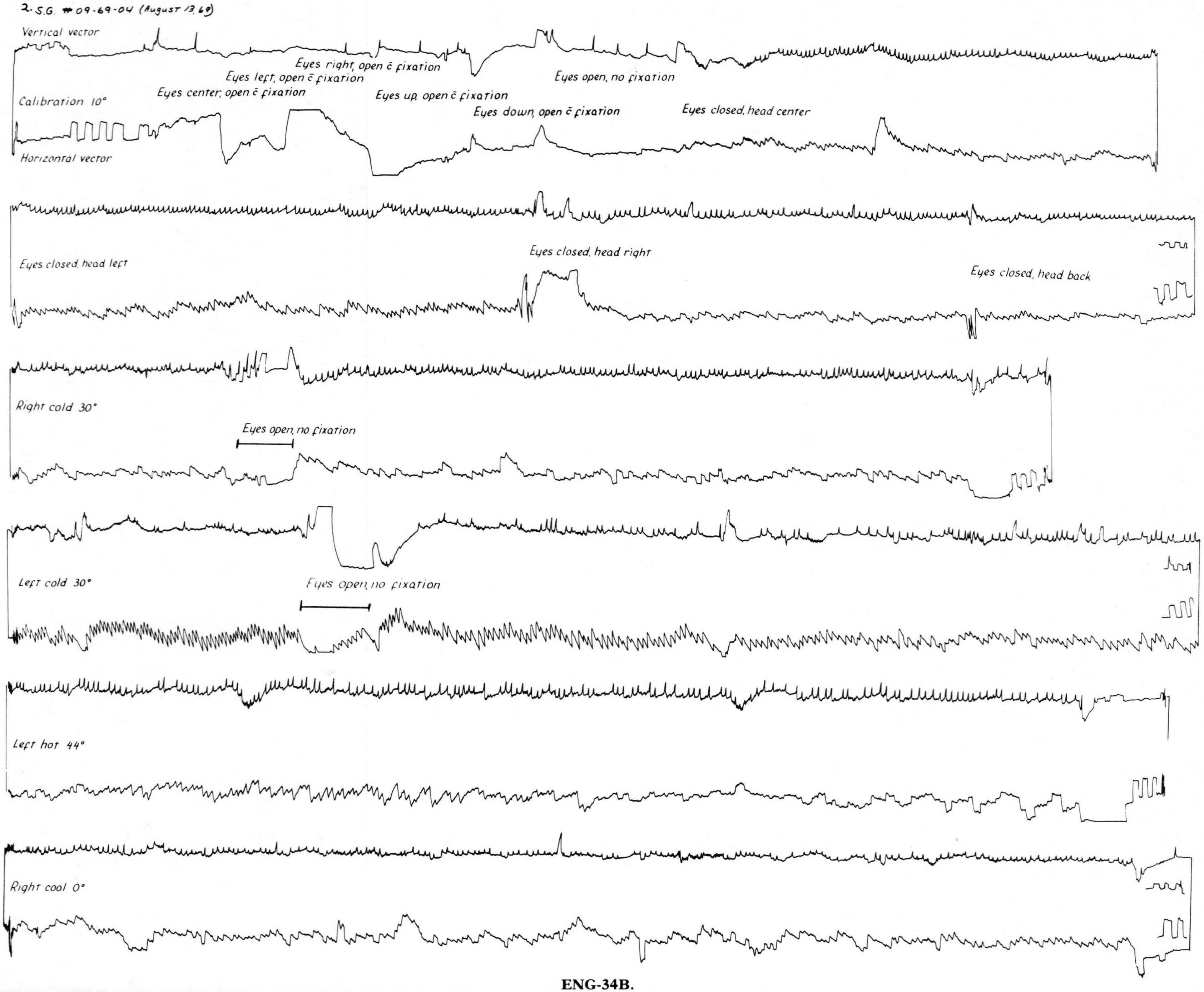

R.S.G. #09·69·04 (August 13'69)

Vertical vector

Calibration 10°

Horizontal vector

Eyes center, open c̄ fixation

Eyes left, open c̄ fixation

Eyes right, open c̄ fixation

Eyes up open c̄ fixation

Eyes down, open c̄ fixation

Eyes open, no fixation

Eyes closed, head center

Eyes closed, head back

Eyes closed head left

Eyes closed head right

Eyes open, no fixation

Right cold 30°

Left cold 30°

Eyes open, no fixation

Left hot 44°

Right cool 0°

ENG-34B.

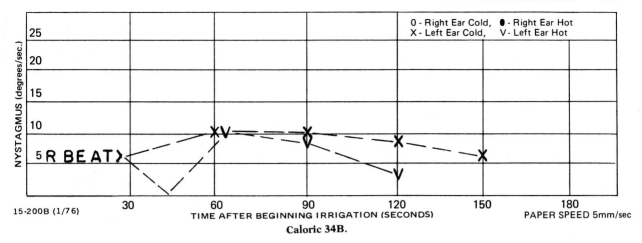

Caloric 34B.

This nystagmus is also now affected by head position, decreasing to near zero in the head-right position.

Bithermal caloric-induced nystagmus still shows a nonresponsive right ear to all stimuli, while those applied to the left ear produced normal responses.

IMPRESSION.   Abnormal examination, spontaneous nystagmus, and nonresponsive right ear.

Diagnosis: Patient was thought to have a possible right cochlear damage secondary to the previous trauma and an early Meniere's disease.

Comment: This case illustrates the importance of serial tracings to further delineate or solidify the impressions gained from a single tracing. This is especially important if an uncertainty exists as to medication influence or if the progress of an acute event is to be followed. In this instance, the patient's past history strongly suggested an old injury. The repeat test indicated otherwise, however.

It should be noted that the spontaneous nystagmus in this case was to the *same* side as the nonresponsive end-organ. This points out that the direction of the spontaneous nystagmus may not indicate the side of the lesion.[15]

The nystagmus that is present during the right ear stimulations is a continuation of the patient's underlying spontaneous nystagmus. This example is clear because the spontaneous rate is unchanged. Others may not be as clear because the tactile stimulus of the water in the ear canal can further arouse the patient, thus producing an apparent increase in the nystagmus. Two clues can be helpful in distinguishing a true caloric response. First, the tactile-induced increase begins immediately, without the usual 30- to 40-second latency for a caloric response. Second, there is no maximum nystagmus at 60 to 90 seconds with tactile stimulation.

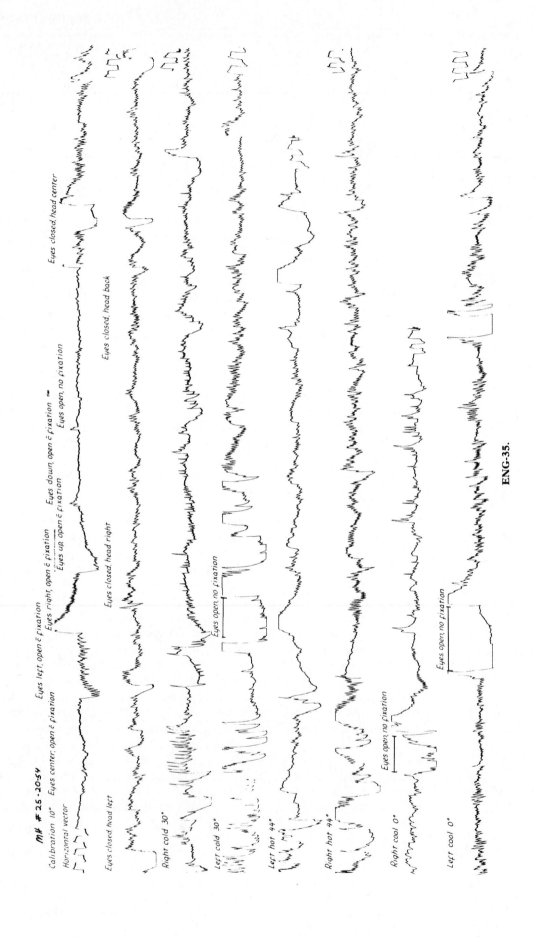

MH # 25-2054

Calibration 10°

Horizontal vector

Eyes center, open c̄ fixation

Eyes left, open c̄ fixation

Eyes right, open c̄ fixation

Eyes down, open c̄ fixation

Eyes up, open c̄ fixation

Eyes open, no fixation

Eyes closed, head center

Eyes closed head left

Eyes closed, head right

Eyes closed, head back

Right cold 30°

Left cold 30°

Eyes open, no fixation

Left hot 44°

Right hot 44°

Eyes open, no fixation

Right cool 0°

Eyes open, no fixation

Left cool 0°

ENG-35.

148

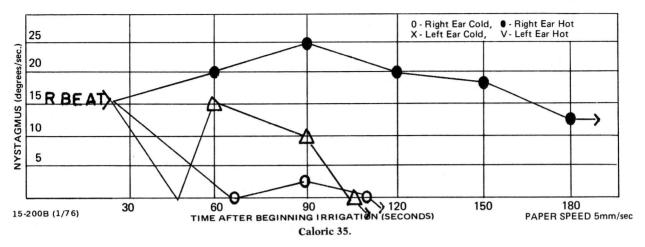

0 - Right Ear Cold, ● - Right Ear Hot
X - Left Ear Cold, V - Left Ear Hot

15-200B (1/76)

TIME AFTER BEGINNING IRRIGATION (SECONDS)

PAPER SPEED 5mm/sec

Caloric 35.

ENG-35

History: A 51-year-old female has had dizziness, not true vertigo, since striking the back of her head on a concrete post 6 months ago. She describes the episodes as similar to being "drunk." She has a long history of left-sided facial and neck pain and of hearing loss in the left ear following childhood otitis media. Irregular eye movements, especially while reading, have been noted previously and labeled congenital fixation nystagmus.

Examination shows bilaterally scarred tympanic membranes with a left myringostapediopexy. There is a right-beating nystagmus with head center and a left-beating nystagmus with left gaze. Left-sided deep tendon reflexes are hypoactive. There is a questionable paresis of the left lateral rectus muscle. Audiogram shows a left combined hearing loss with a 15–30 dB air-bone gap and good discrimination.

ENG Report: Calibration shows a minimal but consistent right overshoot (Fig. ENG-35-1). There is a right-beating spontaneous nystagmus present with the eyes open and vision fixed (see Fig. ENG-35-2), which increases when fixation is prevented and is maximal with the eyes closed (15° per second). This nystagmus is not appreciably affected by head position. There is a bilateral gaze nystagmus, the left lateral gaze being more coarse than the right.

Bithermal caloric-induced nystagmus shows a very hypoactive left ear, only showing a slight response to hot water (it slowed the spontaneous right-beating nystagmus somewhat) and to 5 ml of ice water (it increased the spontaneous right-beating nystagmus about 5° per second). Right ear responses were generally normal when present but did not sustain their activity for the full tracing. There is some dysrhythmia of the caloric nystagmus.

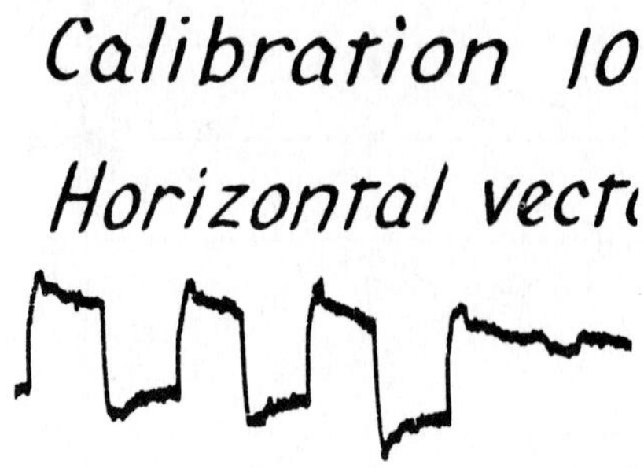

Calibration 10

Horizontal vect

Fig. ENG-35-1.   Segment of calibration tracking.

IMPRESSION.   Abnormal examination, slight tracking overshoot, bilateral gaze nystagmus, spontaneous right-beating nystagmus, and severely hypoactive left ear caloric responses.

Follow-up: The patient was evaluated by a neurosurgeon who performed a lumbar puncture, pneumoencephalogram, and carotid arteriogram. All the tests were reported normal. She presented to the same neurosurgeon 7 years later, complaining of left-sided facial pain and an unchanged examination. Computerized tomography scan was negative.

Comment: This ENG has several characteristics that would lead one to the posterior fossa. First, there is the mild overshoot, primarily to the right, seen in the calibration tracings (Fig. ENG-35-1). (See discussion ENG-17.) Second, the left

Eyes left,

c̄ fixation

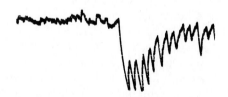

Fig. ENG-35-2.   Transition from eyes center with fixation to left gaze.

gaze nystagmus is a very coarse cerebellar type pattern (right side of Fig. ENG-35-2). (The right gaze nystagmus is very rapid, has lower amplitude, and is probably affected by the spontaneous nystagmus.)

The spontaneous nystagmus shows a classic vestibular pattern: a progressive increase as visual inhibition is removed. Note that the nystagmus is most marked with the eyes closed, reduced with the eyes open without fixation, and even more reduced, but still present, with visual fixation (left side of Fig. ENG-35-2). Such a progression is typical for a lesion somewhere along the vestibular pathway, from end-organ to brain stem. (For a contrasting pattern of visual system nystagmus, see ENG-30.)

There is considerable variation in the slow-phase velocity during positional testing. This is consistent either with swings in level of arousal or (as suspected in this instance) nonspecific brain stem damage.

This woman unquestionably had at least a moderate cerebellar contusion and quite possibly a left labyrinthine injury along with it. Eight years later, she was still having symptoms, and a repeat neurosurgical examination was also negative for a mass lesion.

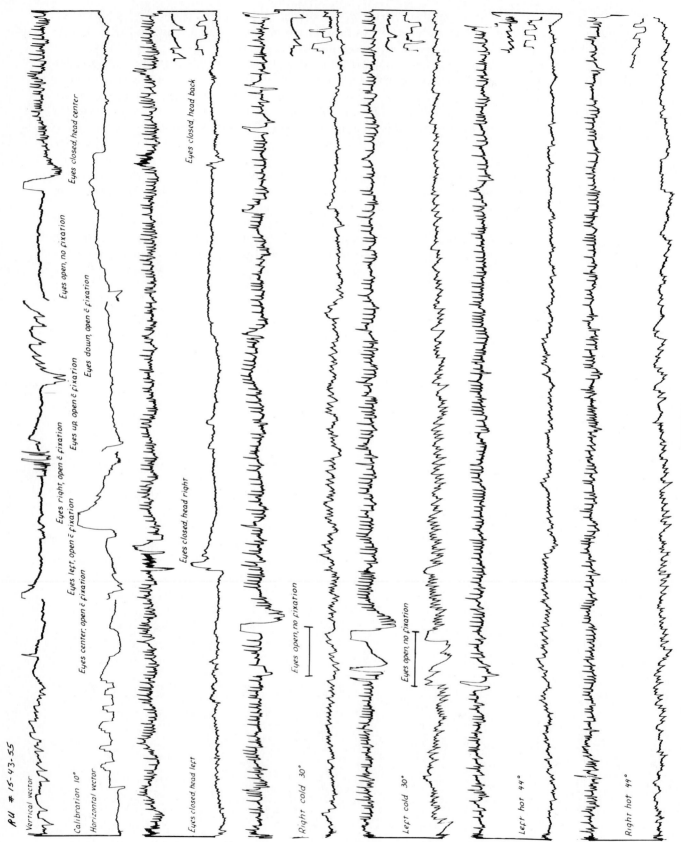

RU # 15-43-55

Vertical vector

Calibration 10°

Horizontal vector

Eyes center, open c̄ fixation

Eyes left, open c̄ fixation

Eyes right, open c̄ fixation

Eyes up, open c̄ fixation

Eyes down, open c̄ fixation

Eyes open, no fixation

Eyes closed, head center

Eyes closed, head back

Eyes closed, head left

Eyes closed, head right

Right cold 30°

Eyes open, no fixation

Left cold 30°

Eyes open, no fixation

Left hot 44°

Right hot 44°

ENG-36.

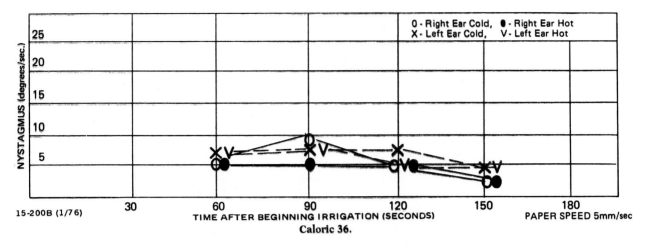

Caloric 36.

ENG-36

History: A 54-year-old male with known metastatic melanoma from the abdomen to the left axilla, right supraclavicular fossa, and base of tongue presents with a 1-day history of faintness, weakness, dizziness, and diplopia. Today, he has developed a slight clumsiness in his right foot. On examination, he has a vertical nystagmus, paresis of the left "internal" (medial?) rectus muscle, and poor conjugate movement of the eyes. A slight hyperreflexia and weakness of the right leg is present. Brain scan and arteriogram show a mass in the left posterior cerebral hemisphere.

ENG Report: There is a calibration tracking abnormality to the right lateral movement (see Fig. ENG-36-1). Vertical calibrations suggest an inability to sustain downward gaze at 10°. There is a borderline right-gaze nystagmus and a down-gaze nystagmus that is of large amplitude. The patient's eyes moved together on calibration tracking, but the abducting eye deviated less than the adducting eye (visual observation). There is no spontaneous nystagmus, but there is a slight right-beating, position-induced nystagmus in the head-left position.

Bithermal caloric-induced nystagmus is generally hypoactive, and the right side appears less responsive than the left. There is a slight nystagmus preponderance to the right.

IMPRESSION. Abnormal examination, abnormal calibration tracking, gaze and position-induced nystagmus, hypoactive right calorics, and slight right-directional preponderance.

Follow-up: The patient subsequently died from cerebral metastases.

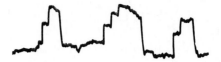

Fig. ENG-36-1.   Horizontal calibration.

Comment: The abnormalities on this ENG are brain stem and posterior fossa defects—not cerebral, where this patient's proven metastasis is located. The calibration abnormality is a form of dysmetria that is usually cerebellar in origin and, unless very prominent, not terribly useful for clinical purposes. Although not provable from the ENG, the most likely explanation for the right-gaze nystagmus is "gaze paresis" in which one or both eyes have a weakly innervated muscle that cannot sustain lateral (or medial) gaze with transient slips toward the center position. Separate eye records would be necessary to prove this contention.

The downward-beating nystagmus is a rare phenomenon (note no indication on the horizontal leads). It occurs from lesions at the level of the oculomotor nuclei and perhaps as far caudally as the upper cervical cord. There is no vertical nystagmus with the eyes closed, only eye blinking.

While there is some indication on this ENG of unusual eye movements, at least half of this information would have been lost if only horizontal electrodes were used. Even with two-channel recording, direct visual observation was more accurate. Intranuclear lesions involving the medial longitudinal fasciculus (MLF) will often not be apparent in any way by routine ENG methods. The ENG reflects only the combined vectors of the movement of both eyes, not individual differences. This is probably the most serious objection to the more general use of ENG techniques by neurologists and neuro-ophthalmologists.[43, 45]

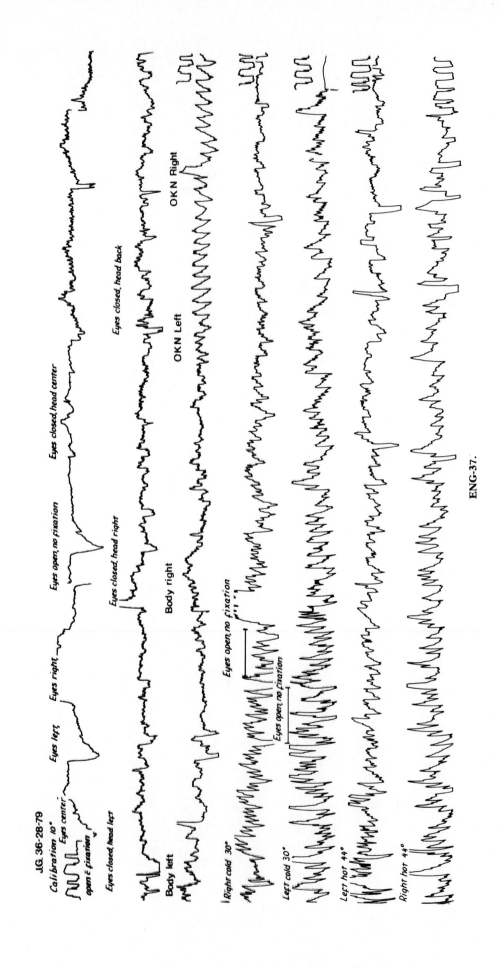

J.G. 36-28-79

Calibration 10°

Eyes center

open & fixation

Eyes closed head left

Eyes left

Eyes right

Eyes open, no fixation

Eyes closed, head left

Eyes closed, head center

Eyes closed, head right

Eyes closed, head back

Body left

Body right

OKN Left

OKN Right

Right cold 30°

Eyes open, no fixation

Eyes open, no fixation

Left cold 30°

Left hot 44°

Right hot 44°

ENG-37.

156

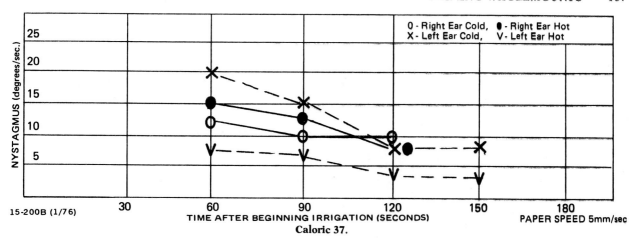

15-200B (1/76)

TIME AFTER BEGINNING IRRIGATION (SECONDS)
Caloric 37.

PAPER SPEED 5mm/sec

ENG-37

History: A 52-year-old male is seen for abnormal movements on the right side. His problems started 20 years ago with a head movement type of tremor which has slowly progressed through the years. Approximately 3 years ago, he noted occasional cramps and jerking movements in the right hand. He underwent full evaluation and was noted to have right facial weakness, twitching of the right facial muscles, right arm incoordination, rigidity, hyperreflexia, and a positive Babinski on the right. His mental status was intact. An earlier extensive workup was negative, but no contrast studies were done.

At the present time, he is unimproved on antiepileptic medications. His mental status is still intact. Exam shows decreased corneal and facial sensation on the right, right hemifacial spasm, right-sided cerebellar signs, loss of fine movement in the right hand, and decreased hearing on the right. The neurologist is very suspicious of a right cerebropontile (CPA) lesion. An arteriogram showed poor opacification of the vertebral basal system and normal carotids. Pneumonencephalogram and posterior fossa myelogram were completely within normal limits.

ENG Report: There is a right- and left-gaze nystagmus that is quite fine in amplitude and which I would attribute to the patient's intention tremor rather than to a cerebellar or visual system defect per se. There is a right-beating spontaneous "nystagmus" of approximately 10°–15° per second that is modestly decreased in the head-left and head-back positions. Total left-right body rotation has no appreciable effect. Optokinetic nystagmus is symmetrical but abnormal (see below).

Bithermal caloric-induced nystagmus is probably within the normal range for velocity, but there is a nystagmus preponderance to the right. There are superimposed eye movements, however, which tend to make an exact measurement difficult. These are probably accentuations of his tremor.

Fig. ENG-37-1. Segment of calibration after the OPN tests.

IMPRESSION.   Abnormal examination; spontaneous nystagmus or tremor affected by head position; abnormal OPN tracking; and right nystagmus preponderance to caloric stimulation.

Follow-up: The patient suffered several myocardial infarctions in the succeeding years and finally died without further progression of his neurological disease.

Comment: This ENG was obtained as part of the patient's examination for a cerebropontile angle lesion, not because of a balance disturbance. The abnormalities are all in the visual system except, possibly, the caloric asymmetry.

There is a defect in pursuit movements. Figure ENG-37-1 shows one defect in the calibration tracking. The eyes do not quite arrive at the target, and a second saccade is required to fix on the light. This tracking error is fairly common in single epochs in normal subjects but is abnormal when consistently present. It is a mild form of cerebellar dysmetria. The dysmetria is more obvious in the OPN tracings (Fig. ENG-37-2). Pursuit to the right is not smooth but regularly irregular. Kornhuber believes this is related to cerebellar cortical degeneration.[27] The end point nystagmus to the left probably has a different anatomic origin but within the cerebellar system.

The presence of a spontaneous nystagmus is debatable. Figure ENG-37-3 shows two segments. There is no fast and slow phase in the first segment. This is abnormal and important, even as an isolated finding, but has no localizing value. In this instance, it is just one more indication that the visual-motor system is defective. It is also an illustration of the need to read the entire tracings, not just selected segments. Also note that there is a delay in onset of at least 15 seconds after the eyes are closed. This is said to be an indication of a CNS defect rather than one at the end-organ or its nerve. One common cause for an onset latency is strabismus.[26]

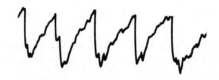

Fig. ENG-37-2. OPN pursuit to the right.

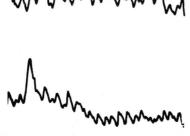

Fig. ENG-37-3. Two segments of eye movement during eyes-closed, head-center testing.

The calculation of the slow-phase velocity of the warm responses would have been in error by being about one-third too fast if the calibrations taken immediately after the calorics had not been used. Note that both of these cause a pen deflection about one-third wider (for 10° of eye movement) than either precaloric calibration or calibration after the right-cool irrigation. The corrected slow-phase velocities were obtained by first calculating the slopes with the conventional overlay and then multiplying by the fractional difference between the normal 10-mm pen deflection and the deflection actually recorded.

ENG-38.

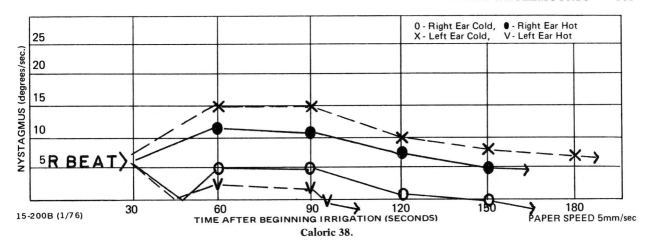

Caloric 38.

ENG-38

History: This 46-year-old male has a 2-year history of monthly episodes of unsteady gait and dizziness associated with vomiting and frontal headaches lasting 1 to 4 hours. He suffered one 12-hour episode of scotomata 2 years ago. In the past 3 weeks, he has noticed a right tinnitus, decreased hearing, and "plugged ear." Examination is normal. There is a right sensorineural hearing loss with a 54-dB SRT, 44 percent discrimination, positive recruitment, and Békésy type I tracking. Internal auditory canal tomograms are normal.

ENG Report: There is no gaze nystagmus. There is a right-beating spontaneous nystagmus that is present with the eyes open without fixation and increases to 5°–8° per second with the eyes closed. It is modestly enhanced in the head-left position.

Bithermal caloric-induced nystagmus responses are asymmetrical, demonstrating a right nystagmus preponderance. This preponderance may have been caused by the superimposition of the above-mentioned spontaneous nystagmus vector upon essentially normal caloric responses.

IMPRESSION. Abnormal examination, spontaneous nystagmus, and asymmetrical caloric responses.

Differential Diagnosis: Meniere's syndrome versus posterior fossa abnormality. Preliminary workup for tumor was negative. Patient's symptoms eventually abated on medical treatment.

Comment: The referring physician was most concerned about a possible posterior fossa defect. The objective findings were more compatible with Meniere's

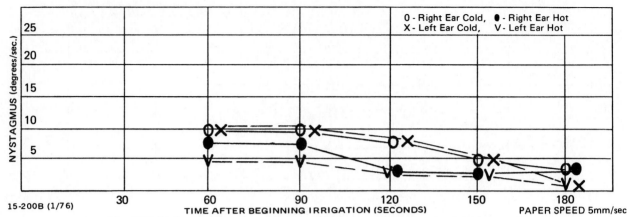

Fig. ENG-38-1. Caloric-induced nystagmus velocities during repeat ENG (see text).

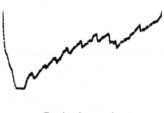

Left lateral

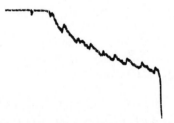

Right lateral

Fig. ENG-38-2. Left and right lateral gaze during repeat ENG (see text).

162

syndrome. A repeat ENG was performed 1 month later and was markedly different from the first (see Figs. ENG-38-1 and ENG-38-2). This second examination showed a bilateral gaze nystagmus, a spontaneous nystagmus only with the eyes open without fixation (never with the eyes closed), and a slight head-left positional nystagmus. Calorics were normal. The presence of a gaze nystagmus in the repeat ENG is a strong enough finding to warrant further workup for a central nervous system problem if a drug effect is ruled out.

These two ENGs offer presumptive evidence for a spontaneous nystagmus affecting caloric responses during the first test. The first examination had a right nystagmus and a right nystagmus preponderance. The second examination had no spontaneous nystagmus (eyes closed) and symmetrical calorics. This relationship between spontaneous nystagmus in nystagmus preponderance is not always true; I am unaware of any firm rules by which to decide when there is and is not a spontaneous nystagmus effect.

Perhaps the most important clinical considerations here are the two quite different ENGs in 1 month. The abnormalities in the first one are quite different than those in the second. This variability is not diagnostic of Meniere's syndrome but is very suggestive. However, a gaze nystagmus and an eyes-open nystagmus on the second ENG are most definitely not compatible with an end-organ defect. Drug effect and/or a minor peripheral visual defect would be important points to check out.

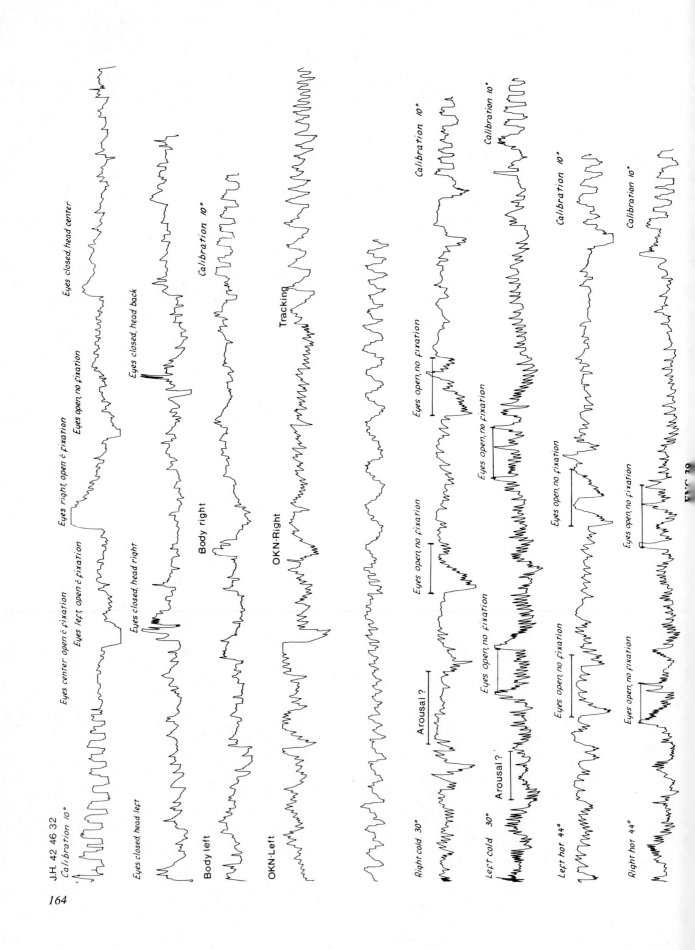

J.H. 42 46 32

FIG. 28

164

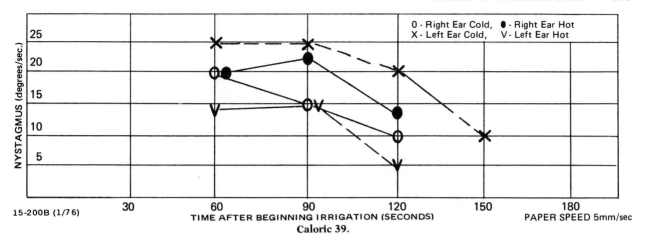

Caloric 39.

ENG-39

History: A 67-year-old male retired mechanic complains that he feels "drunk" intermittently when he rises. This feeling started about 3 years ago after a fall and now occurs about once a week. There is no associated true vertigo, nausea, or vomiting. His wife complains that during the past year he has developed aggressive and argumentative behavior, increased sloppiness, and confusion, with a tendency to become lost. Previous workup included an EEG 3 years ago and a brain scan last year, both of which were normal. Pelvic x-rays show Paget's disease. Examination shows bilateral unsustained gaze nystagmus and poor convergence. Cerebellar testing is normal. His affect is flat, and he has moderate memory loss and inability to abstract. EEG is still normal. Pneumoencephalogram shows diffuse cerebral atrophy with markedly enlarged sulci over the frontal regions.

ENG Report: Calibration is normal. An irregular right- and left-gaze nystagmus is present. There is an intermittent right-beating spontaneous nystagmus present at the approximate rate of 3°–5° per second. This nystagmus is increased with the head rotated to the left. There is no position-induced nystagmus. There is a visual tracking abnormality, especially to the right. He performs adequately when tracking the striped drum but cannot follow a small moving target. There is a question of alertness during testing.

Bithermal caloric-induced nystagmus is within normal limits for nystagmus velocity and right-left symmetry but is dysrhythmic, probably as a result of alertness level.

IMPRESSION. Abnormal examination, possibly abnormal OPN, abnormal tracking, gaze nystagmus, spontaneous nystagmus, and dysrhythmic caloric responses.

Diagnosis: Presenile dementia, possibly Alzheimer's disease, Paget's disease of bone.

Comment: This ENG is one of the more classic in conflicts between real abnormalities and test problems secondary to poor patient cooperation and level of arousal. Even the gaze nystagmus is irregular and intermittent. An intermittent spontaneous nystagmus or one in which there are large changes in either the period or slow-phase velocity as seen here almost always means an arousal problem or a sleepy patient, although there is no way to prove this from these segments of the examination. Level of arousal is probably the basic cause for the poor performance on OPN testing, even though there is a slight asymmetry between the left and right eye movements. Note especially that during the left-going OPN tracing, his eyes make several large drifts from the midplane. This need not be caused by inattention to the task but most commonly is.

Tracking tasks are abnormal, but one can once again be suspicious that the patient is not trying terribly hard to follow the moving light. This test is especially susceptible to arousal artifact and therefore is not very reliable in my experience unless there is a consistent pattern to the eye-tracking defect. None appears here. Benitez, who defined four grades of tracking abnormalities, would probably have classified this one as a type III (definitely pathological).[6] These abnormalities, however, occur in too many other circumstances than simple arousal problems. For example, a high percentage of schizophrenics and some of their relatives also yield highly abnormal tracking patterns.[23]

The best place on an ENG to make judgments on alertness is during the caloric stimulations by comparing the FFS test (eyes-open segments) with the eyes-closed segments. Here the FFS segments are apparently positive during the right-cool stimulation but normal in the other three stimulations. A true FFS positive will demonstrate the effect consistently, not just occasionally. Opening the eyes in these instances served as an alerting stimulus. Note also that there are bursts of nystagmus, then little, and then fairly sizable fluctuations in the slow-phase velocity (left-hot stimulation, for example). These changes are highly suggestive of arousal changes.

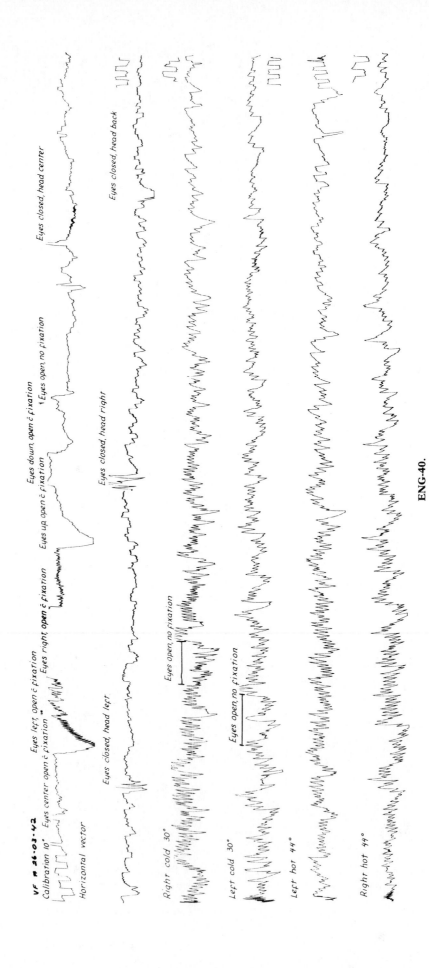

ENG-40.

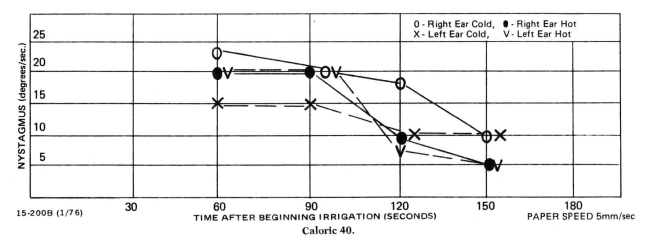

15-200B (1/76)

TIME AFTER BEGINNING IRRIGATION (SECONDS)

PAPER SPEED 5mm/sec

Caloric 40.

ENG-40

History: A 30-year-old female had a 9-year history of progressive dizziness and headache, blurred and double vision, numbness in her right leg, and a staggering gait. In the past 2 weeks, she reports slurred speech and dropping objects inadvertently. Her past medical history includes a "partial hysterectomy" and an oophorectomy. Examination shows a left-beating nystagmus and decreased pain sensation of the right leg. Hearing is normal.

ENG Report: There is a bilateral gaze nystagmus, more marked to the left. There is a slight spontaneous nystagmus beating to the left with a 30-second onset latency and a very slow velocity which is modestly accentuated in the head-right position.

Bithermal caloric-induced nystagmus is symmetrical and within normal limits.

IMPRESSION. Abnormal examination, bilateral gaze nystagmus, slight spontaneous left-beating nystagmus with a latency period and perhaps a positional influence, and normal caloric responses.

Diagnosis: Multiple sclerosis versus Meniere's syndrome by her neurologist. The patient was lost to follow-up but was seen informally (elsewhere) about 5 years later. She was "still" on crutches and in a wheelchair. Her speech was good if she talked slowly.

Comment: The presence of the prominent gaze nystagmus in this patient is very suggestive of central nervous system pathology, but diphenylhydantoin toxicity should be ruled out. Usually, drug-related gaze nystagmus and "cerebellar type" gaze nystagmus has a slower and coarser appearance. This woman's nystagmus is very rapid and is more suggestive of a visual fixation nystagmus than either of the foregoing. In any event, this is clearly not Meniere's syndrome.

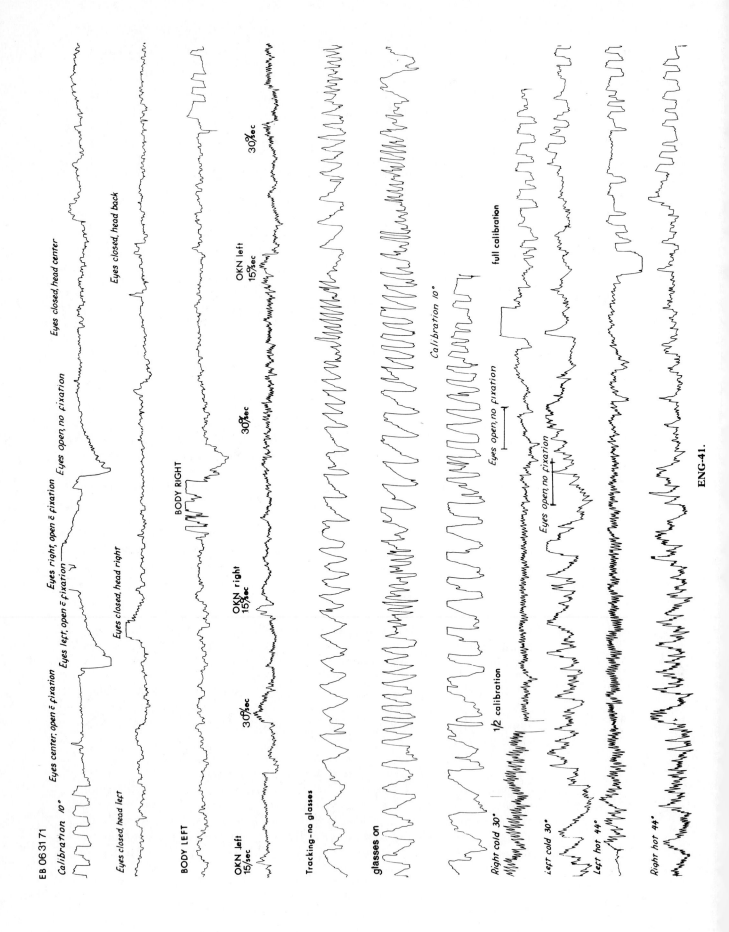

EB 06 31 71

Calibration 10°

Eyes center, open c̄ fixation

Eyes left, open c̄ fixation

Eyes right, open c̄ fixation

Eyes open, no fixation

Eyes closed, head center

Eyes closed, head left

Eyes closed, head right

Eyes closed, head back

BODY LEFT

BODY RIGHT

OKN left
15%/sec

OKN right
15%/sec

OKN right
15%/sec

OKN left
15%/sec

30%/sec

30%/sec

30%/sec

Tracking-no glasses

glasses on

Calibration 10°

Eyes open, no fixation

½ calibration

full calibration

Right cold 30°

Eyes open, no fixation

Left cold 30°

Left hot 44°

Right hot 44°

ENG-41.

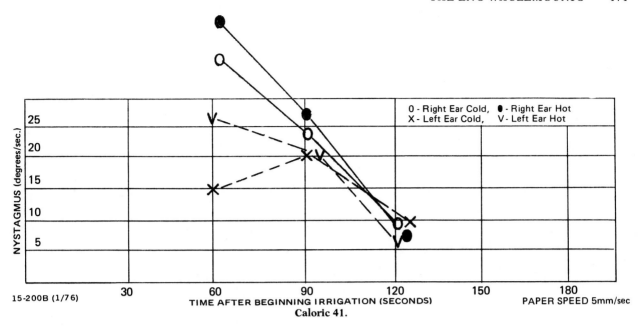

O - Right Ear Cold,   ● - Right Ear Hot
X - Left Ear Cold,   V - Left Ear Hot

NYSTAGMUS (degrees/sec.)

25
20
15
10
5

15-200B (1/76)   30   60   90   120   150   180   PAPER SPEED 5mm/sec
TIME AFTER BEGINNING IRRIGATION (SECONDS)
Caloric 41.

ENG-41

History: This 82-year-old male had successful bilateral cataract surgery several years before he began complaining of a nonspecific constant dizzy sensation. He had some unknown degree of recent left-sided hearing loss. The remainder of his health history and physical status was unknown.

ENG Report: There is no gaze, fixation, spontaneous, or position-induced nystagmus. OPN is asymmetrical in that tracking to the right is at a slightly different vector than tracking to the left. OPN velocities are approximately symmetrical and normal. Tracking of oscillating and sawtooth moving lights is poorly performed and definitely abnormal and is most likely related to poor peripheral vision.

Caloric-induced nystagmus is slightly less on the left but probably still within the range of normal. There is, however, a distinct dysmetria in nystagmus with right-beating nystagmus.

IMPRESSION.   Abnormal examination, poor visual tracking (probably not significant), and nystagmus dysmetria during caloric irrigations.

Comment: This man had 5/200 vision in the right eye and was unmeasurable in his left eye. He was able to follow a visually easy stimulus like the calibration lights and the OPN drum. He failed completely on the more difficult task of tracking an oscillating light source. Poor peripheral vision is one of the common causes for visual tracking errors, and this should be checked if in question, especially when an OPN device other than a large striped drum is employed.

The caloric dysmetria may or may not be significant in an 82-year-old person because of arousal problems or nonspecific cerebral atrophy. I suspect that it is important here, since it is asymmetrical (only to the right) and it would be unlikely that this is a unilateral arousal defect. Very little is known, statistically, about the importance of dysmetria. It is a nonspecific sign which I have observed with posterior fossa, pontine and cerebral lesions, after encephalitis, and with CSF pressure elevation. It can also occur normally in small children.[37]

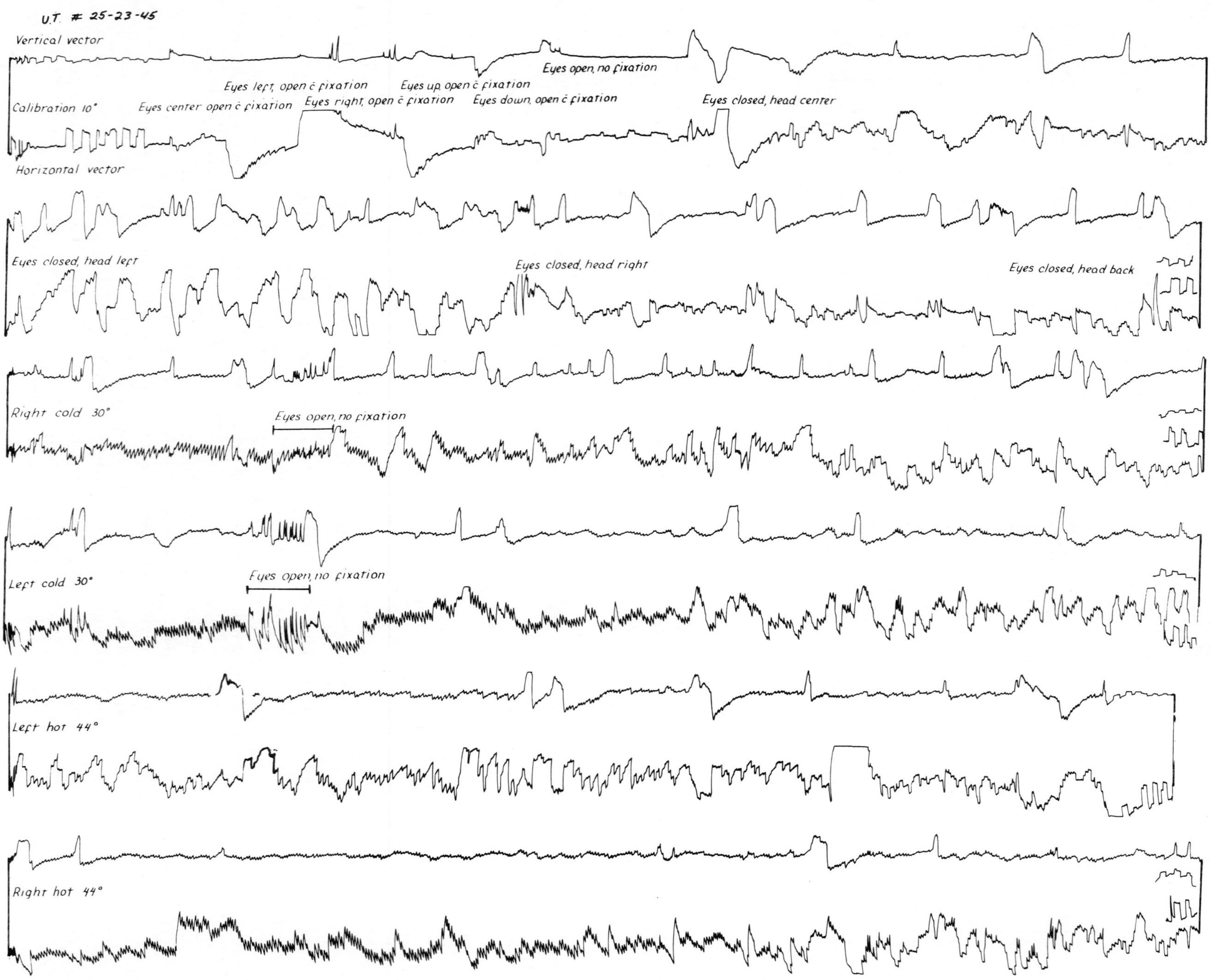

U.T. # 25-23-46

Vertical vector

Calibration 10°

Horizontal vector

Eyes open, no fixation

Eyes closed, head center

Eyes left, open c̄ fixation   Eyes up open c̄ fixation

Eyes center open c̄ fixation   Eyes right, open c̄ fixation   Eyes down, open c̄ fixation

Eyes closed, head back

Eyes closed, head left

Eyes closed, head right

Right cold 30°

Eyes open, no fixation

Left cold 30°

Eyes open, no fixation

Left hot 44°

Right hot 44°

ENG-42.

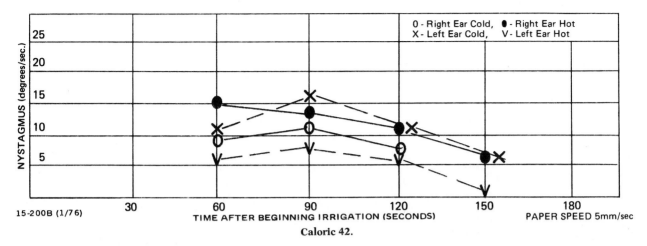

15-200B (1/76)

Caloric 42.

ENG-42

History: A 51-year-old male presents with recurrent sharp, shooting pain over the left third division of the trigeminal nerve. Recently, this pain has become worse and resembles repeated "electric shock" sensations. Dental extractions have not relieved the symptoms. He also recalls transient vertigo beginning 5 years ago and lasting for about 5 minutes. This has recurred perhaps five times since then. He has a subjective right hearing loss unrelated to his vertigo.

Examination shows normal hearing and some hypoesthesia over the left second and third trigeminal divisions. Pneumoencephalogram shows a suspicious density in the left posterior fossa.

ENG Report: Calibration is normal. There is an abnormal gaze nystagmus during right and left lateral gaze (eyes deviated approximately 30° from midline), the left-gaze nystagmus being greater than the right.

There is a right-beating spontaneous nystagmus. Its maximum velocity is highly variable but is approximately 3°–5° per second. There are marked irregularities in the eye motions during positional testing—intermittent large eye position changes with a suggestion of periodicity of 7 to 10 seconds. I do not know the etiology for these or whether they have clinical significance.

Bithermal caloric-induced nystagmus responses are asymmetrical, demonstrating a right directional preponderance, which is probably secondary to the spontaneous nystagmus.

IMPRESSION.   Abnormal examination, abnormal right- and left-gaze nystagmus, a right-beating spontaneous nystagmus unaffected by head position, and asymmetrical caloric-induced nystagmus with a right-directional preponderance.

Diagnosis: Probable trigeminal neuralgia. Follow-up 6 years later shows patient doing well but requiring carbamazepine to control his symptoms.

Comment: This patient's left-gaze nystagmus is definitely pathological, whereas the gaze nystagmus to the right is borderline as to its significance. The large to-and-fro movements seen, particularly during the eyes-closed, head-left position, are called "pendular" movements by some authorities. In this instance, they could probably be considered abnormal, but in the absence of having a specific reason for doing so, they need not be mentioned as pathological in the report.

There is a fair amount of dysrhythmia during the caloric stimulation, especially during the right-hot irrigation, but this is probably within the range of normal inasmuch as most of this dysrhythmia occurs late in the response to caloric stimulation when the stimulus is not as strong.

In retrospect, considering his 6-year relatively normal interval, one might wonder if his pathological gaze nystagmus on the original test might not have been due to medications.

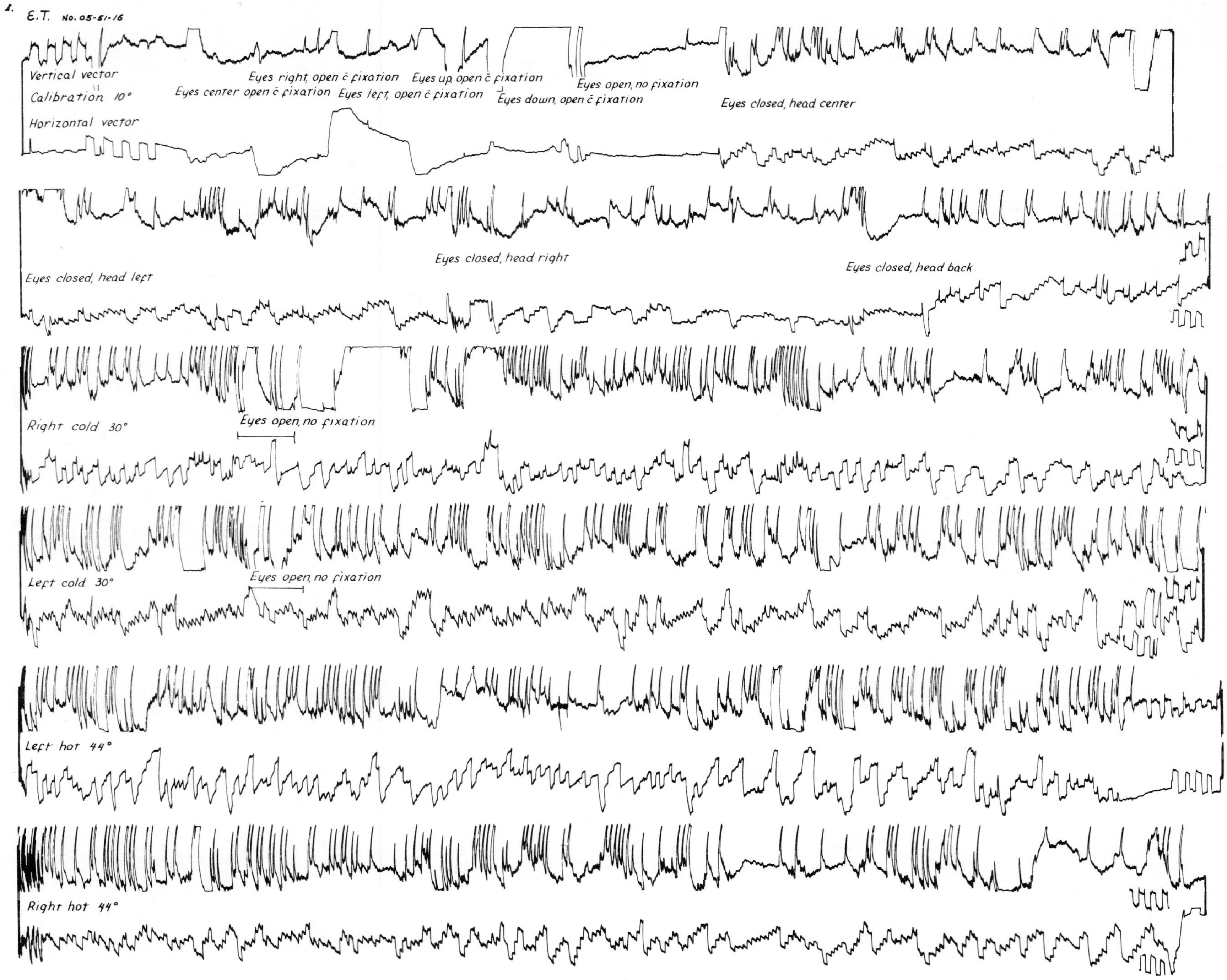

E.T. No. 05-51-16

Vertical vector

Calibration 10°

Horizontal vector

Eyes right, open c̄ fixation   Eyes open, no fixation

Eyes center open c̄ fixation   Eyes left, open c̄ fixation

Eyes up, open c̄ fixation

Eyes down, open c̄ fixation

Eyes closed, head center

Eyes closed, head back

Eyes closed, head left

Eyes closed, head right

Right cold 30°

Eyes open, no fixation

Left cold 30°

Eyes open, no fixation

Left hot 44°

Right hot 44°

ENG-43.

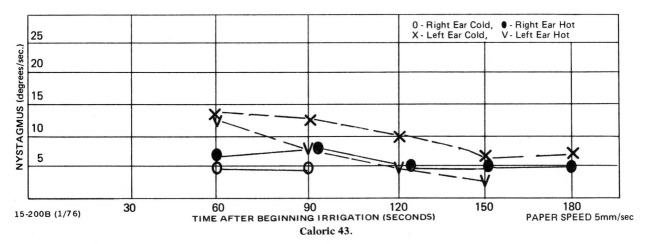

15-200B (1/76)   PAPER SPEED 5mm/sec

TIME AFTER BEGINNING IRRIGATION (SECONDS)

Caloric 43.

ENG-43

History: This 48-year-old female had an acute onset of vertigo and falling to the left, which lasted about 10 hours and was associated with some nausea. There were no auditory symptoms, and the patient felt normal the next day. The second episode occurred 10 days later, with 3 hours of violent vertigo, nausea and vomiting, falling to the left, and "tightness" in both ears. There was no hearing loss, tinnitus, or other neurological symptoms. Examination and audiogram were normal.

ENG Report: There is no gaze or fixation nystagmus. There is considerable blink artifact in the vertical vector channel of this recording. There is an unusual spontaneous nystagmus that beats in two different directions simultaneously. One has an average period of about 0.5 seconds and beats to the right. The other has a longer period of 2 to 3 seconds and beats to the left and upward. The 0.5-second nystagmus is inhibited in the head-right position.

Caloric-induced nystagmus is dysmetric and generally hypoactive. The dysmetria is most prominent in the right-cool and left-warm stimulations—those producing a nystagmus to the left. This dysmetria may possibly be related to the longer-duration spontaneous nystagmus mentioned above. The right calorics are generally more hypoactive than the left.

IMPRESSION. Abnormal examination, unusual spontaneous nystagmus (see above) affected by head position, and hypoactive calorics with dysmetria.

NOTE. Ice water calorics were not done, and these should be obtained if clinically indicated at no cost to the patient.

ADDENDUM. The patient did return for ice water calorics. The dysmetria was still present, but the slow-phase velocities were within normal limits. Final impression: hypoactive calorics with mild dysmetria, cause undetermined.

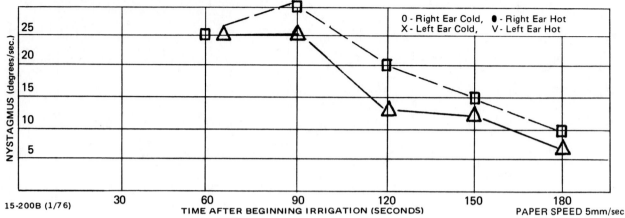

Fig. ENG-43-1.   Caloric responses obtained later using 5 ml of ice water.

Follow-up: The patient continues to have periodic episodes with fluctuation in hearing in both ears at different times. She is controlled on medication. Probable diagnosis is Meniere's syndrome.

Comment: This ENG is an example of caloric nystagmus "recruitment," a phenomenon that occurs in end-organ disorders of the vestibular labyrinth, just as it may in hearing.[28,30] Here, the regular 7°C bithermal calorics were hypoactive, but 0°C stimulations (Fig. ENG-43-1) were normal or near normal. This "recruitment" phenomenon seems to be less consistently present than in hearing recruitment, but possibly only because it is seldom sought.

The dysmetria in the left-beating caloric responses is probably related to the direction conflict with the spontaneous nystagmus beating in the opposite direction.

The spontaneous nystagmus with the near 0.5-second period seems to be a vestibular nystagmus, probably peripheral, because of its modification with head positions. The nystagmus with the slower period (2 to 3 seconds) is beating in a different plane than the vestibular nystagmus—upwards to the left, while the vestibular nystagmus is horizontal. I have no explanation for this most unusual tracing.

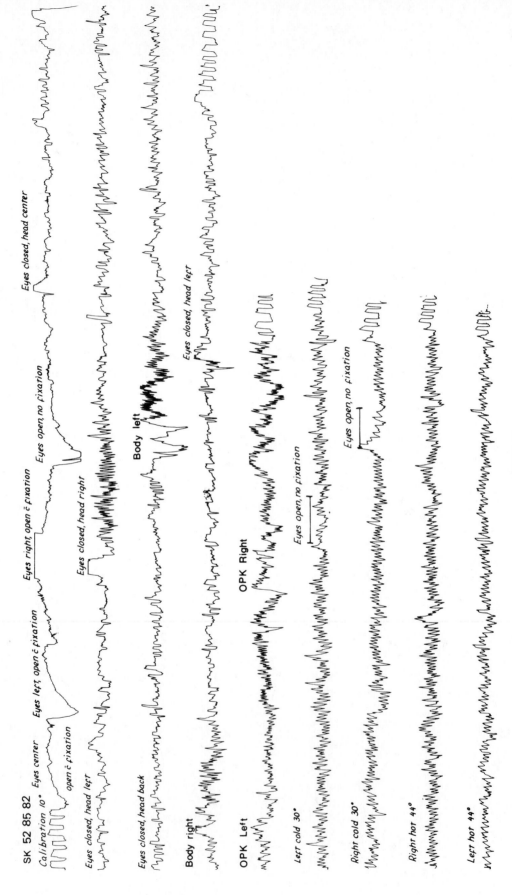

ENG-44.

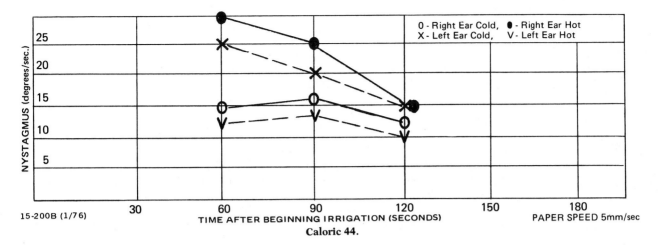

15-200B (1/76)

TIME AFTER BEGINNING IRRIGATION (SECONDS)

PAPER SPEED 5mm/sec

Caloric 44.

ENG-44

History: This 26-year-old male physician has been awakened from sleep for the past 3 nights by severe vertigo and associated nausea. Head motion, especially to the left, increases symptoms. Last evening, he had minimal-to-increasing symptoms upon lying down. Today, he feels slightly out-of-touch with his environment but completely able to carry out his assignments. Six months ago, he had a 1-day episode of vertigo and a right-sided ear fullness associated with an air flight. Otherwise, his history is completely normal. He has had no hearing anomalies.

Physical examination, except for an impressive positional nystagmus, is completely normal. Neurological consultation found nothing else abnormal.

ENG Report: A severe position-induced nystagmus is present, first noted at the beginning of the head-right position (beating at least 30° per second to the right initially, then decreasing over 20 seconds, stopping, then beating to the left at a variable 5° per second, and then eventually decreasing to no nystagmus at about 80 seconds). There was no head-left nystagmus on the first test, but later on there was an equally impressive (30° per second) left-beating nystagmus with total body rotation to the left which also reverted to a slower nystagmus in the opposite direction at about 40 seconds. The intense right nystagmus was again evoked in the body-right position.

IMPRESSION. Abnormal examination; severe direction-changing, position-induced nystagmus; and modest caloric nystagmus preponderance to the right.

Clinical Diagnosis: Multiple sclerosis.

Comment: This is an impressive position-induced, direction-changing nystagmus, especially in a patient who was not particularly symptomatic at the time. The odds for this being the first sign of multiple sclerosis in a healthy 26-year-old are very great. In my experience, a pure positional nystagmus of this magnitude is always caused by a CNS lesion, usually in the posterior fossa. The spontaneous directional change (from right- to left-beating in the head-right position) is unusual but is probably only an "after effect" or "secondary phase" nystagmus.

The odds for a central nervous system cause are also increased in positional nystagmus if the nystagmus beats in the same direction as the head position, that is, right-beating in the head-right position. The odds are about 70 percent in favor of a central cause.

Most direction-changing, position-induced nystagmus is drug-related, and drugs must always be sought. Drug-related nystagmus rarely exceeds a 10° per second velocity, however, except for diphenylhydantoin overdosage.

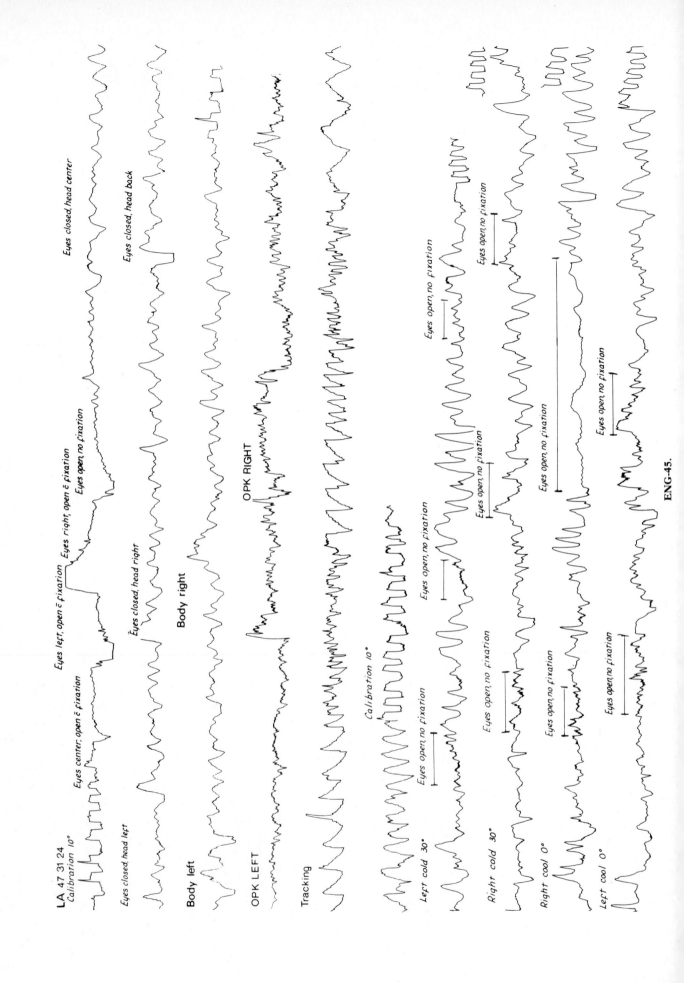

LA 47 31 24

Calibration 10°

Eyes center, open c̄ fixation

Eyes left, open c̄ fixation

Eyes right, open c̄ fixation

Eyes open no fixation

Eyes closed, head center

Eyes closed head left

Eyes closed, head right

Eyes closed, head back

Body left

Body right

OPK LEFT

OPK RIGHT

Tracking

Calibration 10°

Left cold 30°

Eyes open, no fixation

Eyes open, no fixation

Eyes open, no fixation

Right cold 30°

Eyes open, no fixation

Eyes open, no fixation

Eyes open, no fixation

Right cool 0°

Eyes open, no fixation

Eyes open, no fixation

Eyes open, no fixation

Left cool 0°

Eyes open no fixation

Eyes open, no fixation

ENG-45.

ENG-45

History: This 34-year-old female had numerous episodes of dizziness and mental disorientation, all associated with upper respiratory infections over a 3-year period. Three days prior to this ENG, an upper respiratory infection began; a day later she noted dizziness and diplopia, and a friend observed inappropriate conversations with characters on the television. Her hearing was normal. Her Romberg test was positive, and her long tract reflexes were hyperactive. A subsequent neurological examination found minimal ocular dysmetria and poor pursuit movements, disc pallor, difficulty with rapid finger movements on the left, and depressed vibratory sensitivity in the lower extremities.

ENG Report: Calibration trackings are dysmetric and irregular, especially to the right. There is no gaze, spontaneous, or positional nystagmus. During all eyes-closed segments of the test, however, there was a slow and fairly regular "pendular-type" nystagmus. OPN responses are abnormal in both directions, the right slightly worse than the left at some eye speeds.

There is essentially no, or very little, response to caloric stimulation, even with ice water. That which is present is recordable only with the eyes open (failure of visual suppression).

IMPRESSION. Abnormal examination, ocular dysmetria, abnormal OPN tracking, and severely hypoactive calorics with failure of fixation suppression. This is a severe change with increasing abnormalities compared to an examination 2 years ago.

Clinical Diagnosis: Multiple sclerosis.

Comment: The patient had two previous ENGs in the preceding 2 years, both of which were borderline normal and nonspecific. This ENG caught her symptoms and findings in synch. There are numerous positive findings on this tracing. The most striking are the ocular dysmetria, the caloric responses, and the "pendular" nystagmus (also seen in parts of the caloric tests).

The dysmetria is seen best during the OPN tests. She is able to track only one stimulus (slow speed to the left) with any consistency. The breakdown in smooth pursuit at more rapid speeds can also be seen in the ramp-function tracking of the light.

The "pendular" eye movements are rare in our experience. The word "pendular" has been placed in quotes because classical pendular nystagmus is said to occur with the eyes open. It has no localizing value but is a definite CNS abnormality. In eyes-open testing, such a nystagmus is most typically observed in the blind or as a congenital phenomenon thought to originate in the mid-brain.[26]

It is doubtful that the marked attenuation of caloric responses here is actually due to a bilateral peripheral or even eighth nerve lesion. Rather, the vestibular input has been largely and temporarily disconnected from the MLF. Failure of visual suppression of vestibular nystagmus is the final pathological sign here.

None of these findings are specific for multiple sclerosis. There are no specific signs. This ENG, however, coupled with the patient's history of exacerbations during infections, makes any other diagnosis unlikely.

GLOSSARY OF TERMS

There are still some differences in terminology among the several medical specialties which use eye movements and vestibular system tests in clinical diagnosis. The following is a list of these terms as used in this atlas.

AC. Alternating current (*see* impedance).

AMBLYOPIA. In its broadest usage, it means reduced vision without a demonstrable site of lesion. In general usage, it means reduced vision in the nondominant eye of a person with strabismus.

CNS. Central nervous system.

COGWHEELING. An abnormal semiregular interruption of the eyes' smooth pursuit movements by short saccades, typically in the same direction as the pursuit movement. These movements are almost always associated with cerebellar abnormalities.

CONJUGATE EYE MOVEMENTS. Binocular movements in which the eyes move the same distance at the same speed in the same relative planes.

CORNEORETINAL POTENTIAL. The DC or "resting" voltage constantly present between the cornea and the retina. Changes in the actual voltage occur with dark and light adpatation, with retinal degenerations, and with aging.

CPA. Cerebropontine angle.

DC. Direct current, a steady unchanging current.

DIRECTIONAL PREPONDERANCE/NYSTAGMUS PREPONDERANCE. One type of abnormal response to bithermal caloric stimulation of the labyrinth. The nystagmus is more pronounced when beating toward one side than the other; that is, a nystagmus preponderance to the right means that the sum of the slow-phase velocities (or the nystagmus duration) resulting from stimuli normally produce a right-beating nystagmus that is at least 25 percent greater than the sum of the left-beating nystagmus.

ECG. Electrocardiogram.

EEG. Electroencephalogram.

EMG. Electromyogram. In slang usage, it means electrical noise from a muscle contraction.

FAILURE OF FIXATION SUPPRESSION (FFS). An abnormal failure of the visual system to suppress the velocity of caloric-induced vestibular nystagmus.

FFS. *See* failure of fixation suppression.

IMPEDANCE. The resistance to flow of a current when applied voltage is changing; that is , an alternating or AC voltage.

MLF. Medial longitudinal fasciculus.

NYSTAGMUS. Eye movements that are regularly repetitive in any consistent plane or direction (right-left, up-down, tangential, rotary, etc.). There are several "types " of nystagmus which are classified either according to the velocities of the movements (a quick and slow phase, for example) or by the stimulus causing the nystagmus (gaze-induced nystagmus, for example).

Nystagmus, After/secondary. Terms used to describe a normally occurring secondary response to caloric stimulation. This very weak nystagmus beats in the opposite direction from the primary response to stimulation and occurs after the primary response has decayed to baseline.

Nystagmus, Benign positional/vertigo. A special form of transient positional nystagmus in which turning the head to one side, especially with hyperextension (head-hanging maneuver of Hallpike), causes a brisk but transient nystagmus toward that same side.

Nystagmus, fixation. Occurs when the eye is unable to fix and hold focal vision on a target. The waveform of the movements differs according to the cause, which can be in either the sensory or the motor limb of the visual reflexes. Relatively common causes include amblyopia, monocular fixation nystagmus, blindness, spasmus mutans, congenital fixation nystagmus, voluntary movement.

Nystagmus, gaze. This is created by a deviation of the eye from the position of rest. In contrast to fixation nystagmus, visual fixation in the deviated position is not required. Typically, there is a quick phase (a saccade) in the direction of gaze. Relatively common causes include cerebellar defects (most common cause), drugs, internuclear ophthalmoplegias, partial ocular muscle paralysis, physiological causes, high cervical lesions.

Nystagmus, jerk. A commonly used synonym for any nystagmus with a quick and slow phase.

Nystagmus, pendular. This has two quite different forms. In neuro-ophthalmology, the word "pendular" is used to describe nearly all periodic eye movements in which the velocity in both directions is approximately the same, that is, no rapid and slow phases. In the ENG literature, pendular nystagmus is generally reserved for only the very large amplitude, slow period, back-and-forth eye movements seen with the lids closed.

Nystagmus, position-induced. A vestibular nystagmus that appears on moving the head from mid-position. There are two main subtypes, direction fixed and direction changing. In the direction-fixed type (Nylen's type II), head-position changes may cause an increase or decrease in the velocity of the nystagmus, but the vectors always beat in the same plane.[34] In the direction-changing type, the nystagmus beats in one direction in one head position and in the opposite direction in another head position (Nylen's type I).

Nystagmus, positioning. A normal phenomenon wherein a few nystagmus beats occur immediately after a new head position is assumed.

Nystagmus, spontaneous. The term used to describe vestibular nystagmus occurrence when the patient is at rest with the head centered. Small amounts of spontaneous nystagmus occur in normal individuals during ENG recording.

Nystagmus, vestibular. In the broadest sense, it is any nystagmus having a recognizable quick and slow phase not caused by vision. It can be caused by both peripheral (labyrinthine) and central nervous system defects.

OPN/OKN. Optokinetic nystagmus.

OSCILLOPSIA. A subjective sensation of the visual environment caused by defective otolith function, typically bilateral. The person experiences a brief period of visual bouncing with sudden head turning or body jouncing.

PB%. A test for speech discrimination using monosyllables.

PURSUIT MOVEMENT. The eye motion associated with visual tracking of a moving object. The term is also used for eye movement tracking of fixed objects, as in reading a line of print.

SACCADE. The term used for all high-speed eye motion, that is, velocities exceeding at least 100° per second (in brief bursts, speeds up to 700° per second have been recorded). Conceptually, these very rapid movements move the eyes from one visual target to the next. In reading, for example, the saccade occurs between the end of the line above and the beginning of the line below. Saccades are the "fast phase" of a nystagmus beat, the return-toward-center of an optokinetic stimulus, the searchings for a visual fixation point when several visual targets are possible, and a very good index of a person's level of arousal. Abnormalities in these perfectly coordinated, target-oriented eye movements occur at several levels in the visual-motor pathways.

SISI. Short-increment sensitivity index. This hearing test reflects the subject's ability to detect small loudness changes. A high score (about 80 percent) usually reflects an end-organ defect.

TARGET. As used here, it means the object upon which vision is fixed.

TIME CONSTANT. The time required for a steady-state signal to decay to approximately one-third of its initial value. In ENG usage, it is the measure of the low-frequency limit of an AC-coupled strip-chart recorder.

TONE DECAY. A hearing test for unusually rapid adaptation to a steady pure tone stimulus. A positive test usually means a severe loss of nerve fibers in the auditory nerve.

REFERENCES

1. Alexander: Quoted by Jongkees LBW. In Fortscher, Hals- Nas.- Ohrenheilk, 1:1, 1953. (According to Aschan G et al: Acta Otolaryngol, Suppl 129, 1956)

2. Alpert JN: Failure of fixation suppression: A pathologic effect of vision on caloric nystagmus. Neurology 24:891-896, 1974. Coates AC: Central ENG abnormalities. Arch Otolaryngol 92:43-53, 1970. Hart CW: Ocular fixation and the caloric test. Laryngoscope 77:2103-2114, 1967

3. Aschan G, Bergstedt M, Stahle J: Nystagmography. Recording of nystagmus in clinical neuro-otological examinations. Acta Otolaryngol, Suppl 129, 1956

4. Aschan G, Bergstedt M, Stahle J: Nystagmography. Acta Otolaryngol, Suppl 129, 1956

5. Barber HO, Wright G: Positional nystagmus in normals. In Manual of Electronystagmography. St. Louis, CV Mosby, 1976

6. Benitez JT: Eye-tracking and optokinetic tests. Diagnostic significance in peripheral and central vestibular disorders. Laryngoscope 80:834-848, 1970

7. Bos JG, et al: On pathological spontaneous and positional nystagmus. Pract Otorhinolaryngol (Basel) 25:282-290, 1963

8. Bruner A, Norris TW: Age-related changes in caloric nystagmus. Acta Otolaryngol, Suppl 282, 1971

9. Coats AC: Central and peripheral optokinetic asymmetry. Ann Otol Rhinol Laryngol 77:938-948, 1968

10. Coats AC: Electronystagmography. In Bradford LJ (ed): Physiological Measures of the Audio-Vestibular System. New York, Academic Press, 1975

11. Cogan DG: Down-beat nystagmus. Arch Opthalmol 80:757-768, 1968

12. Collins WE: Effects of mental set upon vestibular nystagmus. J Exp Psychol 63:191-197, 1962

13. Collins WE, Guedry FE, Posner JB: Control of caloric nystagmus by manipulating arousal and visual fixation distance. Ann Otol Rhinol Laryngol 71:187-202, 1962

14. Crampton GH: Habituation of vestibular nystagmus. In Bender MB (ed): The Oculomotor System. New York, Harper & Row, 1964

15. Downie DB, Simmons FB: Spontaneous nystagmus direction does not indicate laterality. Arch Otolaryngol 101:358-360, 1975

16. Fitzgerald G, Hallpike CS: Studies in human vestibular function: 1. Observations on the direction preponderance ("nystagmusbereitschaft") of caloric nystagmus resulting from cerebral lesions. Brain 65:115-137, 1942

17. Forssman B: A study of congenital nystagmus, Acta Otolaryngol 57:427-449, 1964

18. Fredrickson JR, Fernandez C: Vestibular disorders in fourth ventricle lesions. Arch Otolaryngol 80:521-540, 1964

19. Gay AJ, Newman NM, Keltner JL, Stroud MH: Eye Movement Disorders. St. Louis, CV Mosby, 1974

20. Hallpike CS: In Wolfson RJ (ed): The Vestibular

System and Its Diseases. Philadelphia, University of Pennsylvania Press, 1966

21. Haring RD, Simmons FB: Cerebellar defects detectable by ENG calibration, Arch Otolaryngol 98:14-17, 1973

22. Harrison MS: Benign positional vertigo. *In* Wolfson RJ (ed): The Vestibular System and Its Diseases. Philadelphia, University of Pennsylvania Press, 1966

23. Holzman PS, Proctor LR, Hughes DW: Eye-tracking patterns in schizophrenia. Science 181:179-181, 1973

24. Jonkees LBW, Maas JPM, Philipszoon AJ: Clinical nystagmography. Pract Otorhinolaryngol 24:65-93, 1962

25. Jonkees LBW: Cervical vertigo. Laryngoscope 79:1473-1484, 1969

26. Jung R, Kornhuber HH: Results of electronystagmography in man: The value of optokinetic, vestibular, and spontaneous nystagmus for neurologic diagnosis and research. *In* Bender MB (ed): The Oculomotor System. New York, Harper & Row, 1964

27. Kornhuber HH (ed): Handbook of Sensory Physiology, Vol. 6, Part 2. Berlin, Springer-Verlag, 1974

28. Litton WB, McCabe BF: Controllable variables in vestibulometry, Arch Otolaryngol 86:445-448, 1967

29. Mattox DE, Simmons FB: Natural history of sudden sensorineural hearing loss, Ann Otol Rhinol Laryngol 86:463-481, 1977

30. Mendel L: Vestibular recruitment in Meniere's disease. Acta Otolaryngol 72:155-164, 1971

31. Miles WR: Modification of the human eye potential by dark and light adaptation. Science, 91:456, 1940

32. Outerbridge JS, Melvill G: Reflex vestibular control of head movement in man. Aerospace Med 42(9):935-940, 1971

33. Nylen CO: Positional nystagmus. J Laryngol 64:295-318, 1950

34. Nylen CO: The oto-neurological diagnosis of tumors of the brain. Acta Otolaryngol, Suppl 33:1-151, 1939

35. Owada K, Shiitse S, Kinura K: The influence of the utricle on nystagmus. Acta Otolaryngol 52:215-220, 1960

36. Pappas DG: The value of including optokinetic nystagmus testing in electronystagmography. Trans Am Acad Ophthalmol Otolaryngol 84:542-548, 1977

37. Riesco-MacClure JS, Stroud MH: Dysrhythmia in the post-caloric nystagmus. Its clinical significance. Laryngoscope 70:697-721, 1960

38. Ruben W: Whiplash with vestibular involvement. Arch Otolaryngol 97:85-87, 1973

39. Simmons FB: Patients with bilateral loss of caloric response. Ann Otol Rhinol Laryngol 82:175-178, 1973

40. Simmons FB, Gillam SF: Frequency response of office ENG machines. Arch Otolaryngol 102:30-32, 1976

41. Spooner TR, Goode RL: The hyperthermic electronystagmogram in multiple sclerosis. Arch Otolaryngol 95:543-546, 1972

42. Stroud MH: The otologist and the midline cerebellar syndrome. Laryngoscope 77:1795, 1967

43. Stroud MH, Newman NM, Keltner JL, Gay AJ: Abducting nystagmus in the medial longitudinal fasciculus (MLF) syndrome. Arch Ophthalmol 92:2-5, 1974

44. Tos M, Adser J, Rosborg J: Horizontal optokinetic nystagmus in cerebral disease. Acta Neurol Scand 48:607-620, 1972

45. Walsh FB, Hoyt WF: Clinical Neuro-ophthalmology, Vol. 1. Baltimore, Williams & Wilkins, 1969

46. Woods WW, Compere WE Jr: Electronystagmography in cervical injuries. Int Surg 51:251-258, 1969

INDEX

Page numbers listed in the index refer to pages of text. ENG numbers listed in the index refer to the ENG wholemounts discussed in Chapter 4. The ENGs listed in boldface type are the more important ones on the topic and are usually discussed in the text of those ENGs. The ENGs listed in roman type indicate that the abnormalities appear in the ENG tracings but are not specifically discussed in the comment sections.

a
b
c
d
e
f
9 g
0 h
1 i
8 2 j